MY SUPERPOWER IS DAD - SURPRISE! IT'S A BOY!

The Complete Super Dad Handbook: Feeding, Diapers, Milestones, Sleep Schedules, and All the Must-Know Baby Stuff You Need to Thrive and Conquer Year 1

Bret Harte

JKKRC Media

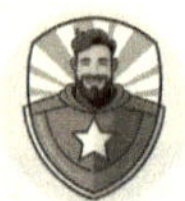

ISBN-13: 9798322334583

For Charlie, My baby baby and destroyer of sleep.
Thanks for the best chaos ever.   Love, Dad

CONTENTS

One and celebrating your journey

PART 1: WELCOME TO THE SUPERHERO LEAGUE

1. THE CALL TO ACTION: THE MOMENT YOU FOUND OUT, THE EMOTIONS, AND THE REALIZATION IT'S REAL

Dude, are you ready for this? Because I still can't fully wrap my head around it, even after months of seeing ultrasound pics and prepping like crazy. I'm about to be a dad. A dad! Seriously, can someone pinch me?

Okay, let's rewind to the day it all hit me. My wife wasn't feeling super great that morning – a little nauseous, some weird cravings. At first, we were brushing it off as just a random bug or something she ate...but then she looked at me with these wide eyes and said, "Maybe we should pick up a pregnancy test, just in case."

Just in case? My heart started pounding. I mean, we'd talked about this – starting a family was definitely the plan, but it felt so far off in some vague, future way. Picking up that little pink box at the drugstore felt like the most surreal mission I'd ever been on.

We decided to do the test together. That bathroom felt like the size of a thimble – nowhere to escape the tension. Those three minutes while we waited were the longest of my life. I kept pacing, fidgeting, trying to crack dumb jokes while my brain turned to mush.

Then, my wife held up the test. Two little blue lines, clear as day. My knees almost buckled. Was I going to pass out? Throw up? I think I actually made some weird choking noise.

In that single instant, a million thoughts and emotions crashed over me like a giant wave:

- Excitement – Holy crap, we're having a baby! I couldn't wipe the goofy grin off my face. I wanted to jump up and down, shout it from the rooftops.
- Fear – Am I ready for this? Can I actually be a good dad? Will I screw this kid up somehow? That little life was suddenly my responsibility.
- Joy – A feeling so deep it brought tears to my eyes. We were building a family, creating this tiny person who would be a part of us. It was mind-blowing.
- Confusion – Okay, now what? My brain went into overdrive, trying to process everything from baby names to whether we needed to

move to a bigger place ASAP.

Those first few hours were a blur. We hugged, we probably cried a bit (hey, no judgment!), and we mostly just stared at each other in shock. It took a while for the news to sink in. Even then, it felt like this amazing, impossible thing happening to *someone else,* not real life.

But as the days turned into weeks, it started to feel real. Seeing that first tiny blob on the ultrasound screen, hearing the heartbeat – like a little galloping horse – that's when the enormity of it all hit me. There's an actual tiny human growing inside of my wife, and I'm going to be his dad.

Suddenly, every dad joke in the book wasn't so cheesy anymore, it was my future. All those dumb action movies where the hero protects his family? They took on a whole new meaning. This wasn't playacting; this was my real-life mission starting right now.

It wasn't all sunshine and rainbows, though. The worry never went away completely. What if something went wrong? Was I financially prepared? Could I handle the sleep deprivation everyone warned me about? Those first-trimester mood swings were, um, challenging (sorry again, babe). There were nights I lay awake, my mind racing, feeling completely in over my head.

But the incredible thing about all of this? Even

though I felt unprepared, even clueless at times, I was already in love with this little dude I hadn't even met yet. That love gave me a strength I didn't know I had.

I started reading every baby book I could get my hands on (the ones I could actually understand, at least). I'd practice swaddling techniques on a teddy bear. We turned our spare room into a half-finished nursery, the walls painted in this calming shade of blue even before we knew we were having a boy. It still felt half-imaginary, but each step made it a tiny bit more real.

The best part, though, was doing it all with my wife. Seeing her belly start to grow, feeling those first little kicks... it deepened our bond in a way I can't describe. We weren't just a couple anymore; we were this team, on the most epic adventure ever.

So yeah, am I completely ready for fatherhood? Probably not. But I'm ready to learn, to figure it out as I go. I'm ready to give this kid all the love I've got and be the best damn dad I can be. Because here's the thing I realized: fatherhood, like any great adventure, isn't about being perfect. It's about showing up, heart open, ready to face whatever comes your way. And that, I can do.

2. SIDEKICKS ASSEMBLE! BUILDING YOUR SUPPORT TEAM – PARTNER, FAMILY, FRIENDS, PROFESSIONALS

Alright, fellow new dad, time to level up your game! I remember when my wife and I found out we were pregnant with our little guy – it was this awesome mix of excitement and the slightest hint of panic. What the heck were we supposed to actually DO with a baby?

The truth is, no one is born knowing everything about parenthood. But one of the best things you can do – for your son, your partner, and yourself – is to assemble your superhero support team. It's about having those people in your corner, ready to offer a helping hand, a listening ear, or just a good laugh when you need it most. So, let's dive into who your most essential sidekicks are and how to build that awesome support squad.

Mission: Partnership – Your Co-Captain in the Chaos

Let's be real, your partner is probably going through her own crazy mix of emotions, and her body's doing some seriously wild stuff. Being a new mom is no joke, and she's going to need you more than ever. So, how do you step up?

- **Communication Central:** Talk openly about your hopes, your worries, even the silly stuff. Those late-night chats when you're both exhausted can be surprisingly helpful in figuring stuff out together.
- **Tag-Team Champions:** There's no point in both of you being sleep-deprived zombies. Figure out a shift system for nighttime feedings and diaper changes so you both get some crucial rest.
- **United Front:** Well-meaning family and friends are bound to give tons of advice, sometimes conflicting. Work with your partner to set some boundaries together about what kind of help you want and when it's time to politely say, "Thanks, but we'll figure this out ourselves."
- **Celebrate the Wins:** Being new parents is hard! Don't forget to acknowledge the amazing things you're both doing, even if it's just

surviving the day.

Mission: Reinforcements – Call in the Grandparents

Okay, let's get one thing straight – grandparents can be total lifesavers in that first year. Whether it's rocking a fussy baby, folding a mountain of laundry, or dropping off a home-cooked meal, they're often bursting with love and eagerness to help. Here's how to make this grandparent power work for you:

- **Know Their Strengths:** Some grandparents are diaper changing ninjas, others are pros at reading bedtime stories. Figure out what they excel at and delegate accordingly.
- **Set Expectations:** Be clear about your needs and boundaries. Do you want an hour of alone time while grandma watches the baby? Do you prefer they call before dropping by? Open communication is key.
- **Don't Sweat the Small Stuff:** Your parents likely did things differently when you were a kid. As long as your baby is safe and loved, try to roll with their way of doing things...sometimes.
- **Appreciation Matters:** A heartfelt thank-you goes a LONG way. Let them know how much their support means to you both.

Mission: Expanding the Squad - Friends, Extended Family & Community

Here's where things get interesting. Think beyond the obvious suspects and get creative with building your support circle:

- **Playdate Posse:** Connect with other new parents. It can be as simple as joining a neighborhood parent group online or hitting up the local playground. There's nothing quite like commiserating with other sleep-deprived dads.
- **The Extended Crew:** Aunts, uncles, cousins – sometimes that extended family network is a goldmine of childcare experience and support. Don't be afraid to ask for help!
- **The Tribe:** Have a close-knit group of friends? Don't forget to lean on them too! Maybe they can bring over takeout, run a few errands, or just offer a listening ear when you need to vent.

Mission: Backup Protocol – When to Call in the Professionals

Sometimes, your usual support team just won't cut it. That's where the professionals come in. Don't be afraid to seek expert help when you're struggling.

- **Pediatricians:** Your baby's doctor is there for way more than just check-ups. They can answer all those nagging questions, address health concerns, and offer developmental guidance.

- **Lactation Consultants:** If breastfeeding is feeling like an impossible riddle, these pros are your secret weapon. They can help with everything from latching issues to supply concerns.

- **Therapists:** Adjusting to parenthood can be emotionally overwhelming for both you and your partner. Individual or couple's therapy can provide a safe space to work through challenges and strengthen your relationship.

- **Sleep Consultants:** When those sleepless nights turn into a full-blown zombie apocalypse, a sleep consultant might be the key to restoring sanity. They can help create a personalized sleep plan for your little one.

The Dad Support Network: Your Online Advantage

Dads, the internet is secretly one of your most powerful tools. Take advantage of these resources:

- **Dad Groups:** Join online communities on Facebook, Reddit, or dad-specific websites. These are great for asking questions, sharing funny stories, and feeling less alone in this new dad world.

- **Reliable Websites:** Trusted sources like the American Academy of Pediatrics (https://www.aap.org/en/) or the Mayo Clinic (https://www.mayoclinic.org/) have tons of evidence-based information on baby care and parenting.

- **Dad Blogs & Vlogs:** Get real-life dad perspectives and inspiration from fellow fathers who share their journeys with a dose of humor.

Listen, being a dad is all about being adaptable. Your support team won't always look the same, and that's okay. The important thing is to know you're not in this alone. So, reach out, ask for help, and embrace the awesome community of parents around you. You got this!

3. GEAR UP: THE ESSENTIAL BABY STUFF (AND WHAT YOU CAN TOTALLY SKIP)

Alright, dads, gear up! Picture this: you brought your little superhero home, and now it feels like your whole house needs an Avengers-level upgrade. Baby stores are overwhelming, online shopping is a maze, and well-meaning relatives keep showing up with gadgets you didn't even know existed.

Don't worry – I've been there. That's why I'm breaking down the baby gear situation like a seasoned mission strategist. We're going to separate the must-haves from the "huh?" items and streamline your base of operations.

Mission Objective: A Functional (and Not Totally Chaotic) Home

Let's be real, babies need a lot of stuff. But they don't need ALL the stuff. Think function over flash. What do you actually need to take care of his basic needs, keep things organized, and inject a little fun?

The Essentials: Your Superhero Starter Pack

- **Safe Sleep Zone:** A crib, bassinet, or pack 'n' play that meets current safety standards is non-negotiable. Get comfy with the guidelines – this is where your little guy will spend a LOT of time. Choose fitted sheets that are snug – no fluffy blankets or pillows as those are safety hazards in that first year.

- **Diaper Duty Command Center:** A changing pad (doesn't need to be fancy), diapers (start with newborn and size 1), wipes, and diaper cream. Stock up, because you'll be amazed how many diapers these tiny humans go through! Pro-tip: set up a small caddy with diaper essentials to take around the house – saves you a million trips.

- **Fueling Station:** Whether you're feeding with bottles, breastfeeding, or a combo, you'll need the right gear. For bottle-feeding, a few different bottle types (babies have preferences!), a bottle brush, and drying rack are essential. Breastfeeding moms might want a comfortable nursing pillow, breast pads, and soothing cream.

- **Mission Control Clothes:** Babies outgrow stuff FAST. Start with comfy onesies, sleepers, socks, and a few warm layers for outings. Think soft, washable fabrics. Skip the adorable-but-impractical outfits...they'll wear them twice before they don't fit.

- **Transport Tech:** A car seat is a legal requirement and a safety essential! Do your research, check the installation, and practice before baby arrives. A stroller is also key for walks, errands, and preserving your sanity.
- **Soothing Arsenal:** A couple of swaddle blankets (the velcro ones are new-dad lifesavers), a few pacifiers (different shapes, just in case), and maybe a white noise machine can really help when your little one is fussing.

Upgrade Options: Consider Your Lifestyle

- **Baby Carrier:** If you're active, this is a game-changer. Skin-to-skin contact is amazing for bonding and gives you hands-free mobility. Choose a style that feels comfortable and secure.
- **Baby Monitor:** Offers peace of mind, especially if your little one sleeps in a separate room. Video monitors are cool, but a simple audio one gets the job done.
- **Swing or Bouncer:** These can be lifesavers for giving you a few minutes to put your feet up while your baby enjoys the gentle motion. Don't feel pressured to get both – one or the other will do.
- **Play Mat/Activity Gym:** Around a few months old, babies start getting more interested in their surroundings. A colorful

mat with some hanging toys gives them a safe place to explore and develops their motor skills.

Stuff You Can Skip (At Least for Now)

- **Wipe Warmer:** Sounds fancy, but babies truly don't care if their wipes are room temperature. Plus, warmers can be a breeding ground for bacteria.
- **Bottle Warmer:** A mug of hot water does the same trick in a pinch. If you're bottle-feeding all the time, then maybe it's worth it, but it's not a day-one necessity.
- **Fancy Changing Table:** You can change a baby on any flat, secure surface. A dresser with a changing pad on top saves space and gives you storage.
- **Tons of Newborn Clothes:** They'll be in and out of those tiny outfits before you know it. Stick to the basics, and accept the hand-me-downs!
- **Complicated Gadgets:** Avoid the stuff with a million features, flashing lights, and weird noises. Babies thrive on simplicity.

The Bottom Line: Build Your Base as You Go

Remember, you don't have to buy everything at once! Focus on the essentials to start with. As you get to know your baby, you'll figure out what additional gear actually makes your life easier.

PART 2: BABY BOOTCAMP – THE BASICS

4. FUELING THE MISSION: BOTTLES, BREASTFEEDING, INTRODUCING SOLIDS – A NO-NONSENSE GUIDE.

Alright, dads, let's get real about feeding our tiny humans. Forget those picture-perfect baby food commercials and visions of happy spoonfuls of oatmeal – this is where things can get messy, confusing, and sometimes a little frustrating. But hey, we're dads, and we figure stuff out!

Bottle Basics 101

Whether you're going all-in on bottles, supplementing, or just want to give your partner a break, let's break down the bottle situation.

- **The Gear:** So many types of bottles! Don't get overwhelmed. Start with a few beginner-friendly ones with simple parts and go from there. And remember, nipple preferences are real – what one baby loves, another might reject. Trial and error is your friend.

- **The Formula Question:** Talk to your pediatrician. They'll help you find the best fit for your little guy, whether that's standard formula, specialty options, or even donor milk.
- **Mixing It Up:** Instructions are there for a reason. Too watery, and your little guy might not get enough nutrients. Too thick, and it could clog the nipple and frustrate him. Follow the directions!
- **Warming It Up:** Most babies like their milk slightly warm, but not hot! Test it on your wrist like you'd test a baby bath. And if you want to invest in a bottle warmer – go for it!
- **The Cleanup:** Those bottles aren't going to wash themselves (sadly). Get a designated bottle brush, dish soap, and a drying rack ready. Hygiene is key for our superheroes-in-training.

Breastfeeding Bootcamp

Dudes, if your partner is breastfeeding, you've got an important support role to play, even if you're not the one actually producing the milk. Here's how you can be a breastfeeding MVP:

- **Become Informed:** Learn the basics – how it works, common challenges, and how long feeds should last. Knowledge is power, and understanding can make a huge difference in helping your partner.

- **The Ultimate Hype Man:** Breastfeeding can be tough, especially in those early weeks. Encouragement and praise go a long way. Tell her she's doing a great job, even on the hard days.
- **Tackle the Logistics:** Grab her snacks, water, a comfy pillow...whatever makes things easier. And when in doubt, offer to do a diaper change or burp the baby to give her a little break.
- **Advocate & Gatekeeper:** Visitors, well-meaning advice, even your own worries – sometimes these things can add extra stress. Be her protector, run interference, and remind her (and yourself!) that she's got this.

Leveling Up: Introducing Solids

Alright, dads, prepare to get a little messy! Around 4-6 months, you'll get the green light to introduce solids. Here's what you need to keep in mind:

- **The Start Line:** It's about exposure, not about meals at first. A few tastes of pureed veggies or baby cereal is a huge deal. The goal is to experiment with flavors and textures.
- **Gag Reflex is Legit:** Don't panic when they gag, it's different from choking. Gagging is a good thing – it means they're learning how to move food around their mouth safely.
- **One at a Time:** Introduce new foods every few days. This makes it easier to spot any potential allergies or sensitivities.

- **Spoon Skills Take Practice:** Patience, dads! More food will probably end up on their face than in their mouth for a while. Don't push it – just make it fun.
- **Finger Foods FTW:** Once they've had some purees AND have that pincer grasp down, you can try soft finger foods. Think well-cooked sweet potato sticks, small pieces of banana, or those melty baby puffs. Always supervise, of course!

The All-Important FAQs

Let's tackle some common questions and worries that crop up on this feeding journey:

- **"How do I know if he's getting enough?"** Wet diapers, weight gain, and meeting milestones are your clues! If you're worried, never hesitate to check in with your pediatrician.
- **"My baby HATES the bottle/purees/any food!"** Don't stress. Take a break, and try again in a few days. Sometimes babies just need time to warm up to new things.
- **"Is it okay to give him water?"** A little bit (a few ounces a day) is usually fine once they start solids, especially in hot weather. But always check with your doc first.
- **"This food thing is expensive!"** You don't have to break the bank on fancy jarred purees. You can make your own by steaming and pureeing veggies or fruits – just make sure

they're cooked super soft.

Remember, dads, feeding is more than just nutrition. It's about bonding, exploring, and starting your little guy on a fun and healthy relationship with food. Don't get bogged down in the details (and definitely don't compare yourself to Pinterest moms!). Relax, have fun, and know that every messy spoonful is a step in the right direction. You're doing awesome!

5. DIAPER DUTY: STRATEGIES, SUPPLIES, AND HANDLING THOSE UNEXPECTED BLOWOUTS

Alright, new dad, I see you looking a little shell-shocked in that diaper aisle. Trust me, I've been there. There are more brands, sizes, and styles than there are Marvel superheroes. But fear not! I'm here to guide you through the...uh, messy side of fatherhood.

Let's start with a truth bomb: Babies poop. A LOT. And those first few poops? Well, let's just say they aren't exactly what you find at the chocolate factory. They change texture and consistency more often than a teenager changes moods. Buckle up because it's about to get real.

The Supplies: Your Diaper-Changing Arsenal

Here's the good news: You don't need a full-on hazmat suit to handle diaper duty. Here's your basic kit:

- **Diapers, Obviously:** Start with newborn size and be prepared to size up fast. Pro tip: Stock up when they're on sale, that kiddo will go through them like Iron Man goes through power cells.
- **Wipes-a-Plenty:** Get the unscented kind for those first few weeks, baby's skin is super sensitive. Later, you can graduate to the fancy ones with all the bells and whistles.
- **Diaper Cream:** A barrier between that tush and the poop-splosion is your best line of defense.
- **Changing Station:** A designated area makes life easier. Just make sure it's safe. Babies are surprisingly wiggly, especially when naked.
- **Distraction Arsenal:** Toys, a goofy song, whatever it takes to keep those little legs from kicking during the mission.

The Techniques: Diaper Changes for Every Situation

Now that you're armed with supplies, let's talk strategy:

- **The Basic Change:** Lay baby down, unstrap the old diaper, marvel for a split second at the creativity of their aim, wipe that little bottom clean (front to back, always!), apply cream, strap on a fresh diaper. It sounds simple, but trust me, practice makes perfect.

- **The "Code Brown" Situation:** You know those moments – the ones where the poop somehow migrates up the back, into the hair, everywhere BUT in the diaper? Deep breaths. Strip baby down, head straight to the sink or tub for a full rinse-down. Sometimes, containment is a lost cause.
- **The Public Change:** The tiny bathroom at the coffee shop was not built for this. Adapt and conquer. Use the stroller, the back of the car, whatever surface you can find. A portable changing pad is your lifesaver here.

Handling the Unexpected: Blowout Tactics

Blowouts are an unfortunate reality when you've got a tiny human powered by milk and puree. Here's how to handle them like a seasoned pro:

- **Damage Control:** Contain the situation as fast as possible. If it's a major eruption, get out of those clothes and into the bath ASAP.
- **Investigation:** Figure out why it happened. Was the diaper too loose? The wrong size? Sometimes it's just bad luck, but identifying patterns can help prevent future leaks.
- **Laundry Hacks:** Poop stains are the worst. Pre-treat with stain remover and wash on hot. Don't be afraid to use the power of the sun – it can work wonders on stubborn stains.

Beyond the Basics: Diapering with Dad Flair

Here's where you get to put your unique spin on fatherhood:

- **Sing Silly Songs:** Diaper changes are the perfect time to let loose with your goofiest tunes. Your baby won't judge your off-key rendition of "Baby Shark."
- **Tickle Time:** Gentle tickles can turn a cranky diaper change into a giggle fest.
- **Make It a Game:** "Peek-a-boo" with the diaper or a race to see who can get the new diaper on faster (spoiler alert: the baby always wins).

The Dad Zone: It's Not All About the Poop

Diaper duty is about more than just keeping your kid clean. It's about bonding too:

- **Skin-to-Skin Time:** Ditch the shirt during changes and let that baby snuggle against you.
- **Eye Contact and Chatting:** Even young babies connect with your voice and expressions.
- **Be Present:** This is your time together. Put the phone down, focus on your little one.

Look, diapers won't always be fun. But they're a part of those precious early moments. Own this dad skill, laugh through the messes, and remember, you're crushing it!

6. LIGHTS OUT: SLEEP STRATEGIES, SCHEDULES, AND HOW TO SURVIVE THE SLEEPLESS NIGHTS

Okay, here we go! Picture me – comfy hoodie, messy dad-bun, and fueled by extra-strong coffee. This chapter is straight from the sleepless trenches, my friend.

Whoa, buddy, get ready because the sleep situation with a newborn is WILD. It's like they haven't gotten the memo that nights are for sleeping. But fear not, fellow dad – we're going to figure this out together.

Phase 1: Understanding the Newborn Sleep Code

Here's the deal: babies operate on a completely different sleep cycle than us. To them, nights and days are a giant blur. Their tiny tummies mean they need to eat often, including in the middle of the night. And let's not forget – they just spent nine months in a cozy, dark womb. It's going to take some adjustment!

The best thing you can do right now is accept the chaos. Don't get hung up on strict schedules or shoulds. Instead, focus on learning your baby's sleepy cues:

- Eye rubbing or staring off into space? He's getting tired.
- Yawning, fussing, or arching his back? It's probably overtired territory.

Catching those cues early and getting him down to sleep will make life easier for everyone.

Phase 2: Building the Sleep Foundation

Once you have a handle on your little guy's sleep signals, we can start working on some helpful routines.

- **The Day/Night Divide:** Help him learn the difference between daytime and nighttime. Keep days bright and active, full of talking and interaction. At night, dim the lights, keep things quiet, and try to avoid too much stimulation.
- **Bath Time Bliss:** A warm bath before bed is super relaxing. Make it part of your nighttime routine followed by snuggles and a bedtime story (even if he can't understand the words yet, the sound of your voice is soothing).
- **Swaddle Up:** Newborns love feeling secure!

A snug swaddle can help calm them down and prevent their little arms from flailing around and waking them up.

- **The White Noise Wonder:** A white noise machine or even just a fan can work miracles. These steady sounds can block out distractions and remind them of the cozy womb environment.

Phase 3: Mastering the Night Shift

Nighttime feedings and diaper changes are inevitable. Here's how to minimize the sleep disruption for everyone:

- **Keep it Low-Key:** No need to turn on all the lights. A soft nightlight will do the trick. Talk softly and keep movements slow and gentle. The goal is to get him fed/changed and back to sleep as quickly and quietly as possible.
- **Tag-Team Tactics:** If you have a partner, work together. Maybe you take the night shift while she gets some solid sleep, then you swap in the morning. Sharing the sleep deprivation load makes it way more manageable.
- **Embrace the Nap:** When baby sleeps during the day, you try to sleep too (I know, easier said than done!). Even a short power nap can boost your energy for round two.

Phase 4: Dealing with Sleepless Night Supervillains

Every baby hits sleep hiccups and regressions. Here's your battle plan for common challenges:

- **The Gas Attack:** All those squirming grunts can be a sign of trapped gas. Try bicycling his legs or doing gentle tummy massage. If gas seems to be a constant issue, talk to your pediatrician.
- **Teething Trouble:** Around 4-6 months, you might start facing the teething monster. Offer a chilled teething ring, try some infant pain reliever (ask your doctor first!), and give extra snuggles.
- **Separation Anxiety Strikes:** As he gets older, he'll become more aware of you leaving. Try a short, consistent bedtime routine to soothe his anxieties.

The Super Dad Survival Kit

This sleep stuff is a marathon, not a sprint. Remember these essentials:

- **Caffeine is your friend:** No shame in an extra coffee (or three).
- **It's okay to ask for help:** Grandparents, friends, a babysitter...anyone who can give you a break so you can catch some ZZZs.
- **Celebrate the Tiny Victories:** The first night he sleeps for a 4-hour stretch? That's a cause for celebration!
- **Laugh whenever possible:** Because

sometimes absurdity is the only way to deal with sleep deprivation.

Dude, you're doing awesome. This newborn stage won't last forever, and those snuggles during sleepless nights? Priceless.

7. BABY BODY MECHANICS: BATHING, DRESSING, NAIL-CLIPPING...WITHOUT CAUSING INJURY

Alright, new dad squad, listen up! Forget those images of dads fumbling with wriggly babies during bath time. I'm here to tell you that baby body mechanics are totally doable – and may even be kinda fun! We're going to ditch the fear and tackle bathing, dressing, and even those ridiculously tiny fingernails like pros.

Bath Time: Not a Shark Tank

First off, I get it. Those early baths can be stressful! Tiny babies are slippery, squirmy, and seem convinced they'll drown in an inch of water. But chill – I've got you covered.

- **Prep Your Battle Station:** Gather everything you need before you start: soft washcloth, baby soap (gentle kind!), towel, clean diaper, fresh clothes. A baby bathtub can help, but your sink works too.

- **Water Temp Check:** Not too hot, not too cold. Aim for lukewarm – test it with your elbow or a baby bath thermometer if you're fancy.
- **Less is More:** We're not cleaning a muddy truck here! A few inches of water is plenty at first.
- **Support is Key:** Use one hand behind his head and neck, and your other hand for washing. Keep your grip secure, but gentle.
- **Start Simple:** Wash face with a damp cloth (no soap), then hair (soap here is okay!), then body. Butt and privates go last – we save the messiest for the end.

Tips from the Trenches

- Babies hate cold air! Keep the room warm and have a cozy towel ready at the finish line.
- Talking or singing keeps baby distracted. Even a bad dad-voice lullaby is better than screams.
- Accidents happen. Don't panic if he pees/poops in the tub, just change the water and keep going. We've all been there.

Dressing the Tiny Human: It's Not Origami

Let's be real, baby clothes are adorable...but putting them on is a puzzle sometimes! Here's how to avoid dressing meltdowns (both yours and his):

- **The Lay-and-Roll:** Start with baby on his back on a soft surface. Onesies go on over the head (gently!). For pants, bunch up the legs and slip them on together like little sausage casings.
- **Button & Snap Strategy:** Do these first! Trying to close buttons on a wiggling baby is pure frustration.
- **Temperature Control:** Babies overheat easily. Layers are your friend! If he feels sweaty, take something off.
- **Comfort is King:** Soft fabrics rule. Scratchy tags are the enemy—cut 'em out!

Nail-Clipping Ninjas

Okay, this one TERRIFIED me at first. Those nails are so tiny! But you gotta do it, or baby turns into a pint-sized Wolverine. Here's the deal:

- **Timing is Everything:** Do it when he's sleepy or right after a bath, when nails are softer.
- **It Takes Two:** Enlist your partner if possible. One person holds baby still, the other does the deed.
- **Tiny Trimmers:** Use baby nail clippers or rounded scissors. Forget regular nail clippers – they're too dangerous.
- **The Pinch Technique:** Gently press the finger pad away from the nail to make clipping easier. Aim for trimming, not a full manicure.
- **Don't Sweat the Quicks:** Accidents happen, and a little bleeding is no biggie. Just apply

a tiny bit of pressure, and give that finger an extra snuggle.

Bonus: Swaddle Like a Pro

Mastering a swaddle is a serious dad superpower. Snuggled babies sleep better! Here's a basic technique:

- **Spread the Love:** Lay the blanket out like a diamond. Fold down the top corner.
- **Baby Placement:** Put baby on top, shoulders lined up with the folded edge.
- **One Side at a Time:** Wrap one side of the blanket across his body and tuck it under him. Same with the other side.
- **Bottom Finish:** Fold up the bottom corner, leaving room for his legs to kick. Wrap remaining side flaps around his body and secure. Not too tight, but snug!

The Dad Zone

Look, baby care can get overwhelming. Here's the thing to remember:

- You're learning as you go. Everyone starts out clueless! Practice makes progress.
- It's okay to ask for help. From your partner, from family, even from those judgy old ladies at the grocery store – they were new moms once too!
- Celebrate the small wins. Nailed a diaper change without getting peed on? That's a

VICTORY, my friend.

Being a dad is an amazing, messy, sometimes scary adventure. Just remember – you've got the instincts, you've got the love, and you've definitely got this!

8. SICKBAY: COMMON ILLNESSES, WHEN TO WORRY, AND YOUR FIRST-AID KIT ESSENTIALS

Babies are little germ magnets. It's like they have a secret mission to collect every single virus and bacteria out there. One day, your little superhero is conquering tummy time, the next, he's got a fever and a nose that sounds like a clogged drain. It's rough seeing your tiny guy feeling under the weather. But don't panic! I'm here to help you navigate the world of sniffles, coughs, and everything that makes your baby just not himself.

The Usual Suspects: Common Baby Illnesses

Here's the lowdown on the most common illnesses your little dude might face:

- **The Common Cold:** The classic. Runny nose, sneezing, maybe a mild fever – sounds familiar, right? This one will probably make a few appearances in year one.

- **Ear Infection:** Super common, especially in babies. Watch out for tugging at ears, crankiness, fever, and trouble sleeping.
- **Stomach Flu:** Fun times ahead (just kidding, this totally sucks). Vomiting, diarrhea, fever, the whole works.
- **Croup:** That scary, barking cough is the tell-tale sign. It sounds worse than it usually is, but definitely needs attention.
- **RSV:** This respiratory virus can be serious for little ones, especially in winter. Look out for wheezing, labored breathing, and lots of mucus.

Warning Signs: When to Call the Pediatrician

Okay, sometimes those little illnesses need more backup than just dad's superpowers. Here's when it's time to call the reinforcements (aka your pediatrician):

- **Fever Under 3 Months:** Any fever in a newborn is a big deal. Call right away.
- **Fever Over 102 F:** A high fever can be a sign of something more serious.
- **Dehydration:** Signs include dry mouth, sunken eyes, and fewer wet diapers than usual. This needs urgent attention.
- **Difficulty Breathing:** Wheezing, fast breathing, or bluish lips mean call the doctor

ASAP.

- **Changes in Behavior:** If your baby is super lethargic, inconsolable, or just acting totally different, it's worth a check-up.

Remember, trust your gut! If something seems off, even if it's not on this list, it's always better to check in with your pediatrician. They're your partners in this crime-fighting gig.

Your Sickbay Arsenal: Stock Up on the Essentials

Being prepared is half the battle. Here's what you need in your first-aid kit:

- **Infant Thermometer:** Rectal temps are most accurate for little ones. Opt for a digital one - it's way easier!
- **Infant Pain Reliever:** Tylenol (acetaminophen) or ibuprofen (after 6 months), but always check dosages with your doc.
- **Saline Nasal Drops:** Loosen up that stuffy nose!
- **Bulb Syringe:** That little blue sucker-outer thing. Perfect for clearing out boogers in a pinch.
- **Humidifier:** Dry air is a cold's best friend, so add some moisture back in.
- **Electrolyte Solution:** For rehydration if your little guy's having tummy troubles. Pedialyte is the classic, but there are other options too.

Extra Supplies for the Dedicated Superhero:

- **Petroleum Jelly:** Perfect for a diaper rash and chapped little noses.
- **Band-Aids:** Because even sick days sometime have boo-boos. Get the ones with fun characters!
- **Small Toys and Books:** Distraction is key when your little one's feeling awful.

Comfort Care 101

Sometimes, the best medicine is just good old-fashioned love and care. Here's how to be an awesome nurse-dad:

- **Cuddles Galore:** Skin-to-skin time is always a win, especially when they're not feeling their best.
- **Hydration Station:** Keep offering liquids, even if it's just small amounts at a time. Breastmilk or formula is ideal if they want it.
- **Popsicle Power:** For sore throats and rehydration, frozen breastmilk or electrolyte pops are a game-changer
- **Peaceful Vibes:** Dim the lights, lower the noise, and make their space a cozy haven.
- **Don't Forget YOU:** Grab a shower, eat a decent meal, and try to tag in your partner whenever you can. You can't help him if you're running on empty.

PART 3: TRACKING HIS SUPER DEVELOPMENT

9. MISSION CONTROL: YOUR BABY'S BRAIN – AMAZING THINGS HAPPENING IN THERE!

Okay, dads, we're about to dive into the most fascinating mission yet: exploring your little dude's incredible mind! I know, I know – right now you're probably thinking about all the spit-up and diaper explosions, which are totally wild too. But trust me, what's happening inside that tiny head is just as awe-inspiring, if not even more so.

Think about it: this little guy is arriving in the world with a brain jam-packed with neurons, just waiting to make connections. During this first year, his brain is going to double in size. Double! That's like upgrading your smartphone's storage in a matter of months. His brain is a supercomputer in the making, and you're right there in the front row as he figures out how to use it.

So, let's learn how this incredible "command

center" operates.

Your Baby's Brain: The Early Days

In those first few weeks, it might not seem like he's doing much besides sleeping, eating, and filling those diapers. But don't be fooled, major construction is happening on the inside! His brain is busy building the foundation for everything he'll learn to do: see, hear, move, talk, and even feel emotions.

Here's a cool fact: he's already forming memories! It's not like he'll remember the details of that epic blowout you cleaned up, but the familiar sounds of your voice, the feeling of your cuddles, all of those are being stored away. Those early experiences shape how his brain wires itself.

The Sensory Superhighway

Your baby's senses are his way of experiencing the world. Think of all those sights, sounds, smells, tastes, and textures as information flooding his brain. At first, it might feel like an overwhelming jumble, but his brain is designed to decode it all.

He might seem fixated on high-contrast patterns, or turn towards familiar voices – that's his brain getting organized. With every sight, sound, and touch, he's building pathways and strengthening connections. These pathways are like superhighways for information, and the more he uses them, the faster and more efficient they become.

From Twitch to Talk: Movement & Milestones

Okay, those first smiles and coos are adorable, but what's actually happening from a brainpower perspective? A ton! As he gains more control over his body – rolling over, sitting up, even those adorable attempts at crawling – he's not just getting stronger, he's also developing his spatial awareness and coordination. His brain is learning to map out his world and how his body fits into it.

And when he reaches for a toy and finally grasps it? That's not just cute, it's a sign of major hand-eye coordination development and problem-solving skills. His brain is saying, "Hey, I see that thing I want, and I figured out how to get it!"

The Language Explosion

Get ready, because that babbling is about to level up! Around six months and onwards, it's like a switch flips. That babbling will start sounding more like actual words, and soon he'll understand what you're saying too.

This is a HUGE deal! His brain is figuring out how language works, that sounds mean specific things, and he can use those sounds himself to communicate. It's the beginning of a whole lifetime of conversations with your little guy.

Your Superhero Role: Fueling the Growth

Okay, dads, I know this all might sound a bit technical, but it's important! Because understanding how his brain works is your key to being the best possible coach for his development. Here's how you can support his amazing brainpower:

- **Be Responsive:** Talk to him, sing to him, read to him, even if he doesn't understand the words yet. The sound of your voice is like rocket fuel for his brain.
- **Playtime Power:** Simple games like peekaboo, stacking blocks, and exploring different textures all stimulate his senses and build those neural pathways.
- **Observe and Adapt:** Don't get fixated on hitting every milestone on a chart. Pay attention to what he's interested in and build your activities around that.
- **Celebrate Every Win:** Whether it's a new word, mastering a skill, or even just a big smile, your enthusiasm builds his confidence and encourages him to keep learning.

From Super Baby to Amazing Kid

Dads, this first year is just the beginning of an awesome journey. His brain will continue to develop at lightning speed, absorbing knowledge, mastering skills, and forming his unique personality. Remember, those everyday moments like bath time, mealtime, and playtime are all opportunities to supercharge his mind. Embrace the adventure, be his biggest cheerleader, and watch in awe as he conquers the world!

10. MILESTONES: WHAT TO EXPECT AND HOW TO ENCOURAGE HIS GROWTH

Get ready for the most exciting journey of your life! Watching your little guy grow and change in that first year is mind-blowing. One minute he's this tiny, squishy bundle, the next he's taking wobbly steps and babbling away. It's incredible!

Before you get caught up in worrying about whether he's "on track," remember this: Every baby develops at his own pace. This chapter isn't about creating a super-baby; it's about understanding what to expect and celebrating his unique progress.

Let's break down the first year month by month, highlighting those awesome milestones to look out for:

Month 1: Hello, World!

- **Super Senses:** His vision is still super blurry, seeing mostly in shades of gray. But don't underestimate him – he can focus on your face from about 8-12 inches away (perfect for those nursing moments!). He'll turn his head towards familiar voices and scents, especially yours and your partner's.

- **Reflex City:** Things are a bit chaotic in the movement department! He has all sorts of reflexes that'll keep you on your toes: a strong grasp reflex (watch those fingers curl around yours!), a rooting reflex (he'll turn his head toward your touch in search of food), and the Moro or 'startle' reflex (where he'll fling his arms and legs out if he feels startled). Don't worry, these start to fade over time.

- **Early Comms:** Crying is his main way of telling you what he needs – hungry, tired, wet diaper, just needing a cuddle. But he's also learning other ways to communicate! Watch for things like smacking his lips when hungry, trying to focus his eyes when he wants to connect, or turning his head away when he's overwhelmed.

How to Help:

- **Skin-to-skin is the best:** Those snuggles aren't just adorable, they help regulate his temperature, breathing, and heart rate. Perfect for both Mom and Dad!

- **Talk it out:** Even though he can't understand your words, he loves the sound of your voice. Narrate your day, sing silly songs – it boosts his language development.

- **Respond to those cries:** It may be exhausting, but responding quickly teaches him that you're there for him. This builds trust and security.
- **Dim the lights:** His eyes are still sensitive, so keep things calm and cozy, especially at bedtime.
- **Swaddle like a pro:** A snug swaddle can mimic the womb, helping him feel secure and sleep better.

Dad Tip: Don't be afraid to get up close. Babies love to study faces, and those early moments of eye contact (even if it's a bit blurry on his end) are bonding magic.

Month 2: Level Up!

- **Head Control:** He's getting stronger! He'll start lifting his head briefly during tummy time. While he might not love tummy time at first, short sessions are vital for building neck and back muscles.
  - **How to Help:** Make tummy time fun! Get down on his level, make eye contact, and sing silly songs. A few minutes a few times a day is better than one long, miserable session.
- **Focus Mode:** He'll track bright objects briefly, and those blurry faces are starting to come into focus a bit more. Faces are fascinating to

babies this age!

- o **How to Help:** Put on a high-contrast black and white patterned shirt. Slowly move your face side to side and up and down while making silly noises. He'll find tracking your face way more interesting! Try dangling brightly colored toys or mobiles just out of reach to encourage those eyes to focus.
- **Social Smile Alert:** Get ready for your first real smile! It'll likely be fleeting at first, but it's the best feeling in the world. These first smiles are often in response to your face and voice.
  - o **How to Help:** Don't underestimate the power of your own goofy faces and funny voices! Talk to him constantly, even if it feels silly at first. Smile and respond to any little coos or gurgles he makes - you're having a whole conversation!

Here's some additional encouragement for dads:

- **Don't Panic:** If your baby isn't hitting every milestone right at the two-month mark, don't stress. Babies have their own timelines, especially those early on. Enjoy these sweet, fuzzy newborn moments!
- **Celebrate the Tiny Wins:** Each little head lift, even a few seconds of focus on a toy, is a huge victory. Celebrate those milestones to keep the positive energy going for both of you.

Month 3: Hello, Interaction

Mini-Gymnast: He'll start kicking more purposefully, and may even be able to roll from tummy to side.

- **The Thrill of Movement:** Get ready for lots of enthusiastic leg kicks! This is him building core strength and discovering the joy of controlling his body. He might not quite have coordinated rolling yet, but these little movements are laying the foundation for those big milestones to come.
- **How to Help:**
  - **Give him legroom:** Dress him in loose-fitting clothes for maximum kick-freedom.
  - **Tummy time galore:** Supervised tummy time on a firm surface helps him build the muscles needed for rolling over.
  - **Dangle enticing toys:** Place a colorful toy just out of reach above him – it'll encourage him to stretch and kick towards it.

Eye Contact Master: Tracking objects gets more refined, and he'll start to focus on and reach for toys.

- **His Vision Sharpens:** He's not just seeing blobs of color anymore! His ability to focus and follow moving objects is getting way better. He'll be fascinated by bright contrasting patterns, and especially by your face.

- **How to Help:**
  - **Slow and steady wins the race:** Move toys slowly across his line of vision to encourage tracking.
  - **Engage his eyes:** Hang a colorful mobile above his crib or play area.
  - **Face-time = Best time:** Talk, smile, and make exaggerated expressions – this is how he learns about the world.

Chatty Baby: He starts cooing and making sweet little vowel sounds – prepare to have full-on 'conversations'.

- **Welcome to Baby Babble:** Get ready for a symphony of coos, gurgles, and adorable squeaks. He's experimenting with his voice and those sweet sounds are his way of 'talking' to you.
- **How to Help:**
  - **Chat back!:** Respond to his coos with enthusiastic babbling of your own. It may feel silly, but it helps him develop communication skills.
  - **Narrate your day:** Talk to him even when you're doing mundane things. "Daddy's changing your diaper now...there you go!" helps him link words and actions.
  - **Storytime:** Reading simple books with big pictures isn't just for future bookworms – it stimulates his language

development even now.

Months 4-6: It's Getting Real!

Rollin', Rollin', Rollin': Somewhere in these months, he'll get the hang of rolling over in both directions.

- **The Joy of Movement:** Rolling over is a HUGE milestone! It's a sign of his growing strength and coordination, and opens up a whole new perspective on the world. He may initially roll by accident, and then get the hang of doing it intentionally.
- **How to Help:**
    - **Roll Model:** Get on the floor and demonstrate rolling yourself (be prepared for adorable giggles).
    - **The Enticement:** Place a favorite toy just out of his reach during tummy time. This encourages him to stretch and use those muscles, potentially leading to that first roll!
    - **Safety First:** Once he starts rolling, never leave him unattended on raised surfaces, even for a second.

Strength Gains: He can hold his head up like a champ and might start pushing up on his arms during tummy time.

- **Mini-Superman:** His neck and core strength

are building rapidly. If he previously hated tummy time, he might start to tolerate it, or even enjoy being able to see the world from this new angle.

- **How to Help:**
  - **Tummy Time Temptations:** Place colorful toys, mirrors, or even your own face in front of him as an incentive to lift up.
  - **Mini-Workout:** Gently roll a big ball under his chest during tummy time – it helps build arm and core strength for future crawling.
  - **Splash Time!:** Bath time is great for building strength. Let him splash and kick – the water provides natural resistance.

Let's Chat: Babbling gets more complex – you might even start to hear "mama" or "dada" sounds (even if he doesn't quite get the meaning yet!)

- **Emerging Language:** His sweet babbles start to turn into chains of sounds like "dadadada" or "mamamama". Get excited, but don't assume he's intentionally calling for you just yet – it's more about playing with sounds.
- **How to Help:**
  - **Imitation Game:** Copy his sounds back to him, adding a tiny variation to expand his repertoire.
  - **Bookworm Beginnings:** Point out and

name objects in picture books. ("See the ball? It's red!")

- ○ **Everyday Narrator:** Talk to him constantly, describing what you're doing, even if it seems basic. This lays the foundation for understanding language.

Months 7-9: On the Move!

Exploration Station: He'll likely master sitting up on his own and maybe even start to crawl or scoot.

- **World, Meet Baby:** Sitting independently gives him a whole new perspective! He can reach toys more easily and has a better vantage point for exploring his surroundings.
- **Mobile Baby Incoming:** Whether it's an army crawl, scooting on his bum, or a more classic hands-and-knees crawl, get ready for a baby on the move! This is exciting but means safety becomes even more crucial.
- **How to Help:**
  - ○ **Safe Play Zone:** Create a designated baby-friendly space with a soft surface and interesting things to explore.
  - ○ **Tempting Targets:** Place toys just out of reach to encourage those first attempts at moving forward.
  - ○ **Obstacle Course Fun:** Pillows and blankets can become a fun, safe way for

him to practice navigating and climbing over things.

- o **Supervise, but Don't Hover:** Let him explore within safe boundaries, but be close at hand in case of tumbles.

Hand-Eye Coordination: Passing toys between hands, banging blocks together – he's discovering what his hands can do.

- **Little Builder:** He's not just grabbing toys anymore; he's manipulating them! Passing objects from hand to hand, banging, and exploring different textures all boost his fine motor skills.
- **How to Help:**
  - o **The Right Tools:** Offer toys of various shapes, sizes, and textures – balls, blocks, rattles, soft books, anything that's safe and interesting.
  - o **Bucket Time:** Give him a bucket and smaller objects to put in and take out – this is a classic for a reason!
  - o **Messy Play:** Once he's into solids, let him explore the texture of food with his fingers. (Be prepared for cleanup!)

Separation Anxiety Alert: He's starting to realize you're separate people – this can mean fussiness when you leave the room.

- **The Emotional Rollercoaster:** Separation anxiety is totally normal. He's starting to understand you can disappear, and he doesn't like it! This can lead to tears and clinging when you try to leave.

- **How to Help:**
  - **Peek-a-Boo Power:** This simple game teaches him object permanence – that you still exist even when he can't see you.
  - **Goodbye Rituals:** Create a quick goodbye routine (a special wave, a kiss) to make leaving more predictable and less scary.
  - **Comfort Items:** A favorite blankie or stuffed animal can offer reassurance when you're not in sight.
  - **Don't Sneak Out:** It may be tempting, but sneaking off intensifies the anxiety. Keep goodbyes short and sweet, but don't disappear without saying anything.

Months 10-12: Little Person Emerging

Almost Walking: He might pull himself to standing, cruise along furniture, or even take those first wobbly steps!

- **Furniture Surfer:** Cruising, where he pulls himself up and walks sideways while holding onto furniture, is a stepping stone to independent walking. Those legs are getting stronger by the day!
- **The Wobbly Wonder:** Those first independent steps are usually hesitant and wide-legged. Be ready with the camera and lots

of excited praise! It's a HUGE deal.

- **Falls Happen:** Prepare for plenty of wobbles and tumbles – it's all part of the process. A soft landing surface and your reassurance help him bounce back.
- **How to Help:**
  - **Safe Exploration:** Make sure furniture is sturdy and remove anything he could pull over on himself.
  - **Push-Along Toys:** Help him practice cruising and gain confidence with a sturdy push toy.
  - **Hands-Off When Possible:** Once he's cruising confidently, try not to hover every second. Let him experience those little wobbles and regain his balance.
  - **Celebrate the Efforts:** Praise every attempt, even if the steps don't quite go anywhere. Your enthusiasm is fuel for his determination.

Pincer Grasp Pro: He can pick up smaller objects using his thumb and forefinger – watch out for choking hazards.

- **Finger Food Fun:** The pincer grasp lets him start self-feeding with small, soft pieces of food! It's a messy, but thrilling, way to explore textures and tastes.
- **Choking Hazard Alert:** Suddenly the whole world looks like a delicious snack – be extra vigilant. Anything small enough to fit through

a toilet paper roll is a potential risk.

- **Exploration Station:** Offer safe, "graspable" objects of various textures and sizes for him to handle and mouth.
- **How to Help:**
  - **Supervise Closely:** Mealtimes and focused playtimes with small objects always require your close attention.
  - **"No Means No":** Be consistent in stopping him from putting non-food items in his mouth. It teaches boundaries and keeps him safe.

Tiny Talker: Babbling gets more defined, and he'll start to understand simple instructions like "no" or "come here."

- **Emerging Words:** Keep an ear out for consistent sounds that seem to be attached to specific things ("dada", "baba" for bottle). These may be his first true words!
- **Receptive Language:** Even if he's not talking much, he's understanding more than you realize. Pointing and naming objects ("Where's your nose?") helps him build vocabulary.
- **How to Help:**
  - **Chatterbox Dad:** Continue talking, singing, and reading to him constantly. The more words he hears, the better!
  - **Follow His Lead:** Pay attention to what he shows interest in and narrate his world. ("Wow, you see the doggy!")

o   **Keep it Simple:** Use short, clear sentences and focused vocabulary to avoid overwhelming him.

11. SUPER SENSES: HOW HE SEES, HEARS, AND EXPERIENCES THE WORLD

Alright, new dad, get ready to have your mind blown. Because here's the thing: your tiny little guy isn't just a bundle of adorable smiles and explosive diapers– he's a sensory explorer! His brain is a sponge, soaking up information from the world around him at an incredible speed. Let's dive into those super senses and see what he's really experiencing.

Sight: From Blurry Shapes to a World of Color

Remember when he was a newborn, and it seemed like he could barely focus his eyes? That was real! Newborns are super nearsighted, seeing things clearly only within about 8-12 inches away -- the perfect distance to gaze lovingly at your face. Over the first few months, his vision sharpens dramatically.

By around three months, he recognizes you! Sure,

it might not be from across the room yet, but give him a big grin up close, and he'll light up. He also starts to love bright colors, contrasting patterns, and anything that moves. Black-and-white toys? Baby genius fuel!

By the end of the first year, your little guy's vision is pretty close to an adult's. He can see detail, track objects like a champ, and explore the world in all its colorful glory.

Sound: Tiny Ears, BIG Listening Skills

Babies are born with their ears fully developed, ready to tune into this noisy world. At first, he might startle easily at loud sounds (who doesn't hate a sudden vacuum cleaner roar?). But don't worry, that sensitivity is normal, and he'll get used to everyday noises in no time.

What's really amazing is how quickly he picks up on language. From day one, he's listening intently to your voice, soaking up patterns and tones. He prefers high-pitched, sing-songy voices (so feel free to get a little goofy when you talk to him). By a few months old, he recognizes his name and turns when he hears it.

Around six months, adorable babbling kicks in– he's practicing those sounds and starting to form his first words. Get excited, because those babbles are the foundation for a lifetime of communication!

Touch, Taste, and Smell: Exploring on Every Level

Your little guy's other senses are equally powerful learning tools:

- **Touch:** His skin is his biggest sensory organ, and he learns SO much through touch. Cuddles, gentle massages, and even exploring different textures (soft blankets, bumpy toys) help him understand his body and the world around him.
- **Taste:** From the first sip of milk to trying out purees, he's constantly bombarded with new flavors. His tastebuds are more sensitive than yours, and his preferences will change rapidly. Don't be discouraged by rejected food – keep offering a variety, and he'll find his favorites.
- **Smell:** While not as strong as an adult's, his sense of smell is essential. He recognizes you by your scent, and the smell of familiar things (like his favorite blanket or your t-shirt) brings him comfort.

Super Dad Tips for Boosting Sensory Development

Now that you understand his amazing senses, how can you make the most of this learning phase? Here are a few fun ways to support his growth:

- **The Narrator:** Describe what you're doing, what he's seeing, or how things feel. "Here's a soft, fluffy ball. Look at the bright red color!"

- **Safe Exploration:** Let him touch and taste (almost) everything. Supervise closely, of course, but giving him room to explore safely builds his understanding of the world.

- **Music Maestro:** Sing songs, play different types of music. Even if he seems unimpressed at first, he's absorbing those sounds and rhythms.

- **Reading Time:** Even before he understands words, looking at colorful picture books together stimulates his sight and starts a love for reading.

- **Follow His Lead:** Observe what he's interested in– a dangling toy, the sound of birds outside. Talk to him about it and let him guide the exploration.

A Note About Sensory Overload

Sometimes, all that sensory input can be too much for him. If he seems fussy, overwhelmed, or looks away, give him a break. A quiet cuddle or a change of scenery can help him reset. It's okay for him (and you!) to need some downtime.

This chapter is a reminder that your little boy is learning constantly, even when it seems like he's just chilling out. By understanding his senses and offering him a rich, stimulating environment, you're giving him an incredible foundation for growth. And that, dad, is a true superpower.

12. LET'S GET PHYSICAL: MOVEMENT MILESTONES – ROLLING, CRAWLING, THOSE FIRST STEPS

Alright, dads, let's get ready to rumble because this chapter is all about those awesome baby moves! Forget sitting still – your little guy is ready to explore, and we're going to be his biggest cheerleaders as he conquers the world (or, you know, the living room carpet).

Rollin', Rollin', Rollin'

It starts with a little wobble, then – BAM! – he's flipping around like a tiny gymnast. Rolling over is a major milestone, marking the start of his journey to independence. Usually, babies get the hang of rolling from belly to back around 4–5 months, and back to belly a couple of months later. But remember, every baby has his own timeline.

Here's the thing: rolling isn't just about moving across the room. It's a big deal for his brain *and* his muscles. It strengthens his core, neck, and arms – all the stuff he'll need for crawling and, eventually, walking. So, how can you give him a little nudge?

- **Tummy Time Power:** This isn't just torture – it's essential! Plop him on his belly for short bursts multiple times a day. Make it fun with toys, songs, and by getting down on his level.
- **Roll Model Behavior:** Get on the floor and show him how to roll. He might look at you like you're crazy, but he's learning!
- **Tempting Targets:** Place a favorite toy just out of reach to encourage him to stretch and roll towards it.

Warning: Once he starts rolling, he won't stop! Never, ever leave your baby unattended on a raised surface – even for a second. This little wiggle worm could surprise you.

The Commando Crawl

Picture this: your baby dragging himself across the floor like a tiny soldier on a mission. That's the classic army crawl, and it usually pops up around 7–10 months. It might look a little goofy at first, but it's a major step towards those wobbly first steps!

Some babies skip the army crawl altogether, opting for scooting on their butts, rolling everywhere, or even a weird crab-walk style. Each style is perfectly fine – it's all about getting mobile! To encourage his crawling quest, try these tactics:

- **The Obstacle Course:** Set up pillows, tunnels, and safe 'roadblocks' to make crawling more interesting. He'll have to maneuver around things – good practice for problem-solving *and* coordination.
- **Follow the Leader:** Crawl across the room in front of him, encouraging him to copy you. Make it a silly game with lots of smiles and encouragement.
- **The Treasure Hunt:** Hide a favorite toy where he has to crawl to get it. Motivation is key!

Remember, some babies take a little longer to crawl. Don't compare him to other kids; just focus on having fun and celebrating his progress when it happens.

Cruisin' For a Bruisin'?

Once he's got crawling down, get ready for the next move: pulling up to stand! Around 9-12 months, he'll start using furniture, your legs, or anything sturdy to hoist himself up. Now, this is where things get both exciting *and* a little nerve-wracking.

Cruising – walking sideways while holding onto stuff – is how he practices balance and builds walking muscles. Here's what you can do:

- **Babyproof Like a Pro:** Pad sharp corners, anchor furniture to the wall, and lock away anything hazardous within reach. Your once-tidy house might look like a padded cell, but safety first!

- **Push the Pace:** Get him a push toy designed for early walkers. This gives him something sturdy to hold onto as he practices his moves.
- **High Fives All Around:** Lots of cheering and praise when he pulls up, cruises, or takes those wobbly steps. Your excitement is his fuel!

Those First Steps...and Falls

There's no feeling quite like seeing your child take those first hesitant steps. It's a heart-stopping, tear-jerking moment. But let's be real; there will *also* be plenty of tumbles along the way. Most babies start walking sometime between 9 and 15 months, but there's a wide range of normal.

Here's the deal: trying to force him to walk before he's ready won't work. It's about his development, not you pushing the timeline. Focus on these things instead:

- **Barefoot is Best:** Let those little feet feel the ground for better balance and sensory input. Socks can actually make him slip!
- **Stumbles are Learning:** Don't freak out with every fall. Minor bumps and bruises are part of the process.
- **Celebrate Every Effort:** Whether it's one step or a few wobbles across the room, make him feel like a champion.

The Joy of Movement

This whole movement milestone thing is amazing to watch, but there's more to it than meets the eye. Think about it – he's learning how his body works, gaining confidence, and starting to explore the world on his own terms. That's powerful stuff!

So, dads, let's ditch the sidelines and get involved:

- **Playtime Gets Physical:** Roughhouse a little (safely!), chase him around, and dance like nobody's watching. Movement should be fun!
- **Outdoor Adventures:** Take him to the park, let him crawl on the grass, and explore different textures. Variety is key for his development.
- **Document the Journey:** Take videos, photos, and write down those milestone moments. This is a year you'll want to remember.

Remember, every baby moves at his own pace. Don't get caught up in comparing him to other kids or stressing about exact timelines. Your job is simple: cheer him on, help him feel safe, and celebrate the incredible journey of his first year on the move!

13. COMMUNICATION STATION: BABBLING, GESTURES, AND THOSE MAGICAL FIRST WORDS

Let's get real for a minute. I'm not going to sugarcoat it — being a dad can be amazing, but it can also feel pretty overwhelming. I mean, you have this tiny human relying on you for everything! Sometimes my brain goes into overdrive, worrying if I'm messing this whole thing up.

I'm betting I'm not the only dad who's felt this way. Whether it's a nagging worry about doing the right thing or a full-on panic attack in the baby aisle at Target, it's okay to admit these anxieties are real. It doesn't make you a bad dad; it makes you human.

Here's the thing to remember: You're not alone. Let's break down some of the most common dad anxieties and figure out ways to combat them.

Fear #1: "I'm going to break him!"

Those first few weeks, I was terrified of holding my son. What if I dropped him? What if his neck wasn't supported enough? Turns out, babies are way tougher than they look. With a little practice, handling him got less scary.

Here's what helped me:

- **Start slow:** Support his head and neck during those early days. If you're nervous, practice on a pillow or stuffed animal first.
- **Watch how others do it:** Your partner, mom, grandma – anyone with experience can show you the ropes, boosting your confidence. (There are also a ton of baby care videos online.)
- **Remember, it's okay to ask for help!** Putting him down gently and asking for backup is way better than trying to handle something when you're feeling unsure.

Fear #2: "I'm not providing enough."

Especially if your partner is breastfeeding, it's easy to feel a little useless in the milk department. But dads can provide in a million other ways! My wife and I got into a groove where I'd handle bath time, burping, and diaper changes, giving her a chance to rest and actually focus on feeding.

What can you do?

- **Be her rock:** Ask what she needs, whether

it's a snack, a break, or just some words of encouragement. Supporting her supports the baby!

- **Own some tasks:** Find the things you enjoy doing with your little guy and make them your 'specialties'. It could be playtime, reading, or just those adorable post-bath snuggles.
- **Remember, bonding isn't just about feeding:** Your presence, your touch, even just talking to him with a silly voice provides comfort and security.

Fear #3: "What if I can't protect him?"

The world can feel like a scary place, especially when you're looking at it through the eyes of a dad. I remember this wave of worry hitting me when we'd take our son out for the first time. What if we got in an accident? What if he got sick? What if something terrible happened and I couldn't stop it?

Taking a deep breath is key here. Here's how I manage those protective-dad instincts:

- **Learn the basics:** Look up baby first aid, CPR, and safety practices. Feeling prepared boosts your confidence.
- **Be proactive, not paranoid:** Do things like babyproofing your home and researching safe car seats. Taking action turns worry into responsible planning.
- **Focus on what you CAN control:** You can

control giving him a loving home, keeping him healthy, and teaching him about the world. That's huge!

Fear #4: "I don't have any idea what I'm doing!"

Imposter syndrome is a real thing, and it hits dads too. Some days I look at my son, then back at myself, and think, "They seriously let me take this kid home? I haven't got a clue!"

It's important to remember none of us were born knowing how to be a dad. Here's the good news:

- **Everyone's learning as they go:** Even those dads who seem super confident are figuring it out alongside you.
- **Ask for help, without shame:** Your partner, friends, family, pediatrician – they all have valuable knowledge to share.
- **Resources are your friend:** There are tons of dad-focused blogs, websites, and organizations. Find your online community – knowing you're not alone is powerful.

The Big-Picture Takeaway

Anxiety is a normal part of fatherhood, but it doesn't have to define you. Remember these key points:

- **Be patient with yourself:** Learning to be a dad is like learning any new skill – it takes time and practice. Cut yourself some slack!

- **Celebrate the wins:** Every diaper change, every smile you coax out, every milestone – it's all worth celebrating.
- **Humor is your superpower:** There will be days when all you can do is laugh at the absurdity of it all. Embrace the messy, imperfect side of parenting.
- **Reach out when you need to:** There's no shame in reaching out for help. Whether it's talking to your partner, a friend, or seeking professional support, remember taking care of yourself makes you an even better dad.

You might feel a bit overwhelmed right now, but I promise you, those early anxieties will fade a bit with each passing day. That feeling of "I don't know what I'm doing" will gradually be replaced with "Hey, I'm actually getting the hang of this!"

And before you know it, you'll be the one guiding a confused, nervous new dad, passing on your hard-earned wisdom that, yes, handling a newborn IS a little scary, but absolutely worth the adventure.

PART 4: SUPER DAD, SUPER SELF

14. YOUR KRYPTONITE: COMMON DAD ANXIETIES AND HOW TO DEAL

Let's get real for a minute. I'm not going to sugarcoat it — being a dad can be amazing, but it can also feel pretty overwhelming. I mean, you have this tiny human relying on you for everything! Sometimes my brain goes into overdrive, worrying if I'm messing this whole thing up.

I'm betting I'm not the only dad who's felt this way. Whether it's a nagging worry about doing the right thing or a full-on panic attack in the baby aisle at Target, it's okay to admit these anxieties are real. It doesn't make you a bad dad; it makes you human.

Here's the thing to remember: You're not alone. Let's break down some of the most common dad anxieties and figure out ways to combat them.

Fear #1: "I'm going to break him!"

Those first few weeks, I was terrified of holding my son. What if I dropped him? What if his neck wasn't supported enough? Turns out, babies are way tougher than they look. With a little practice, handling him got less scary.

Here's what helped me:

- **Start slow:** Support his head and neck during those early days. If you're nervous, practice on a pillow or stuffed animal first.
- **Watch how others do it:** Your partner, mom, grandma – anyone with experience can show you the ropes, boosting your confidence. (There are also a ton of baby care videos online.)
- **Remember, it's okay to ask for help!** Putting him down gently and asking for backup is way better than trying to handle something when you're feeling unsure.

Fear #2: "I'm not providing enough."

Especially if your partner is breastfeeding, it's easy to feel a little useless in the milk department. But dads can provide in a million other ways! My wife and I got into a groove where I'd handle bath time, burping, and diaper changes, giving her a chance to rest and actually focus on feeding.

What can you do?

- **Be her rock:** Ask what she needs, whether

it's a snack, a break, or just some words of encouragement. Supporting her supports the baby!

- **Own some tasks:** Find the things you enjoy doing with your little guy and make them your 'specialties'. It could be playtime, reading, or just those adorable post-bath snuggles.
- **Remember, bonding isn't just about feeding:** Your presence, your touch, even just talking to him with a silly voice provides comfort and security.

Fear #3: "What if I can't protect him?"

The world can feel like a scary place, especially when you're looking at it through the eyes of a dad. I remember this wave of worry hitting me when we'd take our son out for the first time. What if we got in an accident? What if he got sick? What if something terrible happened and I couldn't stop it?

Taking a deep breath is key here. Here's how I manage those protective-dad instincts:

- **Learn the basics:** Look up baby first aid, CPR, and safety practices. Feeling prepared boosts your confidence.
- **Be proactive, not paranoid:** Do things like babyproofing your home and researching safe car seats. Taking action turns worry into responsible planning.
- **Focus on what you CAN control:** You can

control giving him a loving home, keeping him healthy, and teaching him about the world. That's huge!

Fear #4: "I don't have any idea what I'm doing!"

Imposter syndrome is a real thing, and it hits dads too. Some days I look at my son, then back at myself, and think, "They seriously let me take this kid home? I haven't got a clue!"

It's important to remember none of us were born knowing how to be a dad. Here's the good news:

- **Everyone's learning as they go:** Even those dads who seem super confident are figuring it out alongside you.
- **Ask for help, without shame:** Your partner, friends, family, pediatrician – they all have valuable knowledge to share.
- **Resources are your friend:** There are tons of dad-focused blogs, websites, and organizations. Find your online community – knowing you're not alone is powerful.

The Big-Picture Takeaway

Anxiety is a normal part of fatherhood, but it doesn't have to define you. Remember these key points:

- **Be patient with yourself:** Learning to be a dad is like learning any new skill – it takes time and practice. Cut yourself some slack!

- **Celebrate the wins:** Every diaper change, every smile you coax out, every milestone – it's all worth celebrating.
- **Humor is your superpower:** There will be days when all you can do is laugh at the absurdity of it all. Embrace the messy, imperfect side of parenting.
- **Reach out when you need to:** There's no shame in reaching out for help. Whether it's talking to your partner, a friend, or seeking professional support, remember taking care of yourself makes you an even better dad.

You might feel a bit overwhelmed right now, but I promise you, those early anxieties will fade a bit with each passing day. That feeling of "I don't know what I'm doing" will gradually be replaced with "Hey, I'm actually getting the hang of this!"

And before you know it, you'll be the one guiding a confused, nervous new dad, passing on your hard-earned wisdom that, yes, handling a newborn IS a little scary, but absolutely worth the adventure.

15. MAINTAINING THE SECRET IDENTITY: BALANCING FATHERHOOD WITH YOUR OTHER ROLES

Let's be honest – becoming a dad is like suddenly becoming a superhero. But guess what? You don't get to leave your Clark Kent identity behind. You've still got work, maybe a social life (what's that?), and all those other parts of you that existed before this tiny human showed up.

Figuring out how to balance being a rockstar dad with all your other responsibilities can feel like juggling chainsaws...while blindfolded. But it's possible, I promise!

Here's how to maintain your secret identity without losing your mind:

Work-Life Balance: Mission Possible

Whether you're heading back to the office or working from home, there's going to be an adjustment period. Here's some survival tips:

- **Communicate with your boss (if you have one):** Be upfront about any schedule changes, and negotiate flexibility if possible. Remember, showing your commitment as a dad doesn't diminish your commitment to your work.
- **Set boundaries:** When your workday is over, try to actually switch off. Easier said than done, I know, but those emails can often wait. Your son needs your focus in the present.
- **Adjust your expectations:** You might have to scale back those late nights at the office, at least for a while. It's okay to say "no" to extra work and focus on quality over quantity.

Don't Let Your Friendships Fade

Remember those guys you used to hang out with? Yeah, they probably miss you. Maintaining those friendships is important, but it takes extra effort with a baby in the picture. Try these strategies:

- **Schedule it:** Make time for a phone call or occasional hangout, even if it's just for an hour. Putting it on the calendar makes it more likely to happen.
- **Invite them over:** Sometimes it's easier to bring your friends into your new world than to try to escape to theirs. Backyard BBQ with the baby napping? Game night where your little guy is the adorable distraction? Get creative!

- **Be honest:** If you're exhausted and can't make that late-night concert, don't feel guilty. True friends will understand.

Keeping the Romance Alive

Your relationship with your partner is going to transform. It has to. You're teammates in this parenting game, and communication is key. Here's some advice:

- **Tag-team approach:** Don't fall into the traditional roles of one parent always being "on duty." Take turns, share the load, and give each other breaks.
- **Schedule time for just the two of you:** Even if it's just a walk after the baby's asleep, having those moments to reconnect as a couple – not just as parents – is essential.
- **Don't forget the little things:** A sweet text, a silly inside joke, leaving a note on the bathroom mirror – keep up those gestures that show you still see and love each other.

And Finally, Don't Forget About YOU

I know, it sounds crazy when you barely have time for a shower. But neglecting self-care is a recipe for a grumpy, burnt-out dad. Here's how to sneak in some "me-time":

- **Embrace the small moments:** That commute? Prime podcast time. Waiting at the doctor's office? Catch up on a chapter of that book you've been meaning to read.

- **Get moving:** Even a quick workout session boosts your mood and energy. Bonus points if you can involve the baby – stroller walk, anyone?
- **Say "yes" to help:** When someone offers to babysit, take them up on it. Do something that recharges you, even if it's just taking a nap!

The Truth? It WON'T Be Perfectly Balanced

Some days you'll feel like you're crushing this whole multi-tasking thing. Other days you'll drop all the balls at once. That's normal. Just remember, being a dad doesn't mean your life has to stop – it just means you get to bring your amazing little sidekick along for the ride!

16. RECHARGE THE BATTERIES: SELF-CARE ESSENTIALS FOR DADS (IT'S NOT SELFISH!)

Okay, let's address the elephant in the room: Dad burnout is real! Between the sleepless nights, endless diaper changes, and constant demands on your attention, it's easy to feel completely drained. You might be tempted to put your own needs on permanent hold, thinking that's what makes a good dad.

But here's the thing: You can't be the best dad when you're running on empty. Think of it like your phone – when the battery's dead, nothing works properly! Self-care isn't selfish; it's essential for being the awesome dad you want to be.

Why Does Dad Self-Care Matter?

- **Better energy, better dad:** When you're rested and taking care of yourself, you have more energy and patience for all those awesome (and exhausting) dad duties.

- **Stronger relationships:** Irritability and stress can strain your relationship with your partner. Taking care of yourself actually benefits your whole family.
- **Role modeling for the future:** Want your son to grow up understanding the importance of well-being? Show him what it looks like by taking care of yourself.

The Self-Care Toolkit: Practical Strategies

Okay, I know you don't have time for day-long spa retreats. So, let's focus on quick, realistic self-care wins:

- **Prioritize the basics:** Sleep (as much as possible!), healthy food, and some form of movement. Even a short walk around the block can do wonders for your mood.
- **The 10-Minute Reset:** When you're feeling overwhelmed, take a dedicated 10 minutes. Meditate, listen to your favorite music, or just stare at the ceiling – anything that helps you de-stress.
- **Tap your support system:** Ask your partner, parents, or friends for help so you can take some guilt-free "me time."
- **Rediscover your hobbies:** What did you enjoy before the baby arrived? Schedule little pockets of time for those, even if it's just 20 minutes of reading or playing a video game.
- **The 'No Guilt' Zone:** Stop feeling bad for

taking care of yourself. Think of it as investing in your ability to be an amazing father.

Busting Dad Self-Care Myths

Myth 1: "Real dads tough it out." Nope! Toughing it out leads to burnout. Prioritizing well-being makes you a stronger, better dad in the long run.

- **The Superhero Trap:** Society sometimes tells dads to suppress their emotions and just power through. But the truth is, bottled-up stress and exhaustion makes you less patient, less present, and more likely to snap under pressure.
- **Strong ≠ Emotionless:** True strength includes admitting you need support sometimes. Taking care of yourself physically and mentally isn't a weakness – it's the responsible thing for both you and your family.
- **Leading by Example:** Kids learn by watching. Showing your son that it's okay to prioritize wellbeing sets a healthy example he'll carry with him for life.

Myth 2: "I don't have time." Even 5 minutes of self-care can make a big difference. Build it into your routine, not just when you're on the verge of collapse.

- **The "All or Nothing" Fallacy:** You don't need hours at the spa to practice self-care. The goal is to build small, sustainable habits into your day.

- **Small Wins Add Up:** A 5-minute walk around the block to clear your head, a quick stretch while the baby naps, or just three deep breaths when you're feeling overwhelmed – all of this matters.
- **Prevention > Cure:** Don't wait until you're at the breaking point to think about self-care. Make it a regular part of your routine, like brushing your teeth.

Myth 3: "Self-care costs money." Many of the best self-care practices are free or low-cost: going for walks in nature, chatting with friends, or learning relaxation techniques online.

- **Budget-Friendly Doesn't Mean Less Effective:** Sure, fancy gym memberships and retreats are nice, but not essential. The core of self-care isn't about spending, it's about intention.
- **Get Creative:** Think about things you genuinely enjoy that also reset you. Is it playing music for 10 minutes? Kicking a ball around with your kid? Building something in the garage? Those count!
- **Free Resources:** There's a ton of free content online – guided meditations, workout videos, even dad groups for support and connection. Libraries are also a great resource!

The Bottom Line

Remember, dad, you're not just a superhero for your son; you're a role model. Showing him that it's okay (and important!) to take care of yourself gives him a powerful lesson for life. So give yourself permission to fill your own cup, and you'll find you have even more to give.

17. MISSION: BONDING WITH YOUR BABY BOY – PLAYTIME IDEAS AND BEYOND

Okay, dads, I know life can feel like a blur those first few months. Diapers, feeds, spit-up – it's easy to get caught in the routine and miss out on the fun part. But here's the thing: Bonding with your little guy is not only awesome, it's crucial for his development and your own happiness as a dad.

Forget about those complicated play setups you see on Instagram. Bonding can happen in simple, everyday moments. Let's break it down:

Power Up Your Daily Routine

- **Narrate your world:** Talk to him constantly, even when it feels a little silly. Describe what you're doing, the colors you see, the funny sounds you hear. This builds his language skills and makes him feel included.
- **Turn chores into playtime:** Diaper

change? Make it a tickle fest! Give him a running commentary as you get him dressed. Bathtime? Time for splashy songs and silly faces!

- **Babywearing for the win:** Strap him into a carrier or sling while you do stuff around the house. Feeling your closeness is comforting, and it frees up your hands for a much-needed coffee break.

Level Up With Playtime

- **Face time is the best time:** Get down on his level, make funny faces, stick out your tongue. Nothing sparks more giggles than a goofy dad!
- **Explore his senses:** He's learning through touch, sight, and sound. Give him different textures to feel, show him brightly colored toys, play music, and sing (no matter how badly!).
- **Reading rocks, even for babies:** Don't worry about finishing a whole book. Point out pictures, name shapes, and make up your own silly stories as you go.
- **Tummy time adventures:** Make tummy time fun by placing interesting toys just out of reach, or get down beside him for some eye-to-eye connection.

Beyond Play - Connection is Everywhere

- **Snuggles aren't just for Mom:** Make skin-to-skin contact a priority. Hold him close and let him feel your warmth and heartbeat.

- **Take over the soothing:** Babies need comfort as much as they need food. Figure out what soothes him – rocking, singing, a gentle walk – and become his go-to for calming those cries.
- **Look into those eyes:** It might sound cheesy, but eye contact is powerful. Hold his gaze, smile, and let him know he's the most important thing in your world.

Dad Pro-Tips:

- **Don't be afraid to experiment:** Babies change quickly, so what worked last week might not fly today. Keep trying new things!
- **Follow his lead:** If he's interested, awesome! If he's getting fussy, take a break. You want bonding to be fun for both of you.
- **Your vibe matters:** Babies pick up on your mood. If you're stressed, it's okay to hand him off and recharge. Coming back relaxed makes for better bonding time.

Dads, remember there's no one "right" way to do this. The more present you are, the stronger your bond will grow. And trust me, nothing beats those first laughs, those big gummy smiles, and knowing that YOU made those happen. This is where the real superhero stuff begins.

18. THE PARTNER PROTOCOL: KEEPING YOUR RELATIONSHIP STRONG THROUGH THE CHANGES

Okay, let's address the elephant in the room: having a baby changes EVERYTHING. Not just in your life, but also in your relationship with your partner. Suddenly, you're not just a couple; you're a sleep-deprived, slightly-panicked parenting team. And let's be honest, sometimes the romance takes a backseat to spilled milk and marathon diaper changes.

I'm not going to lie, it's easy to feel disconnected after your little guy arrives. Those late-night chats have turned into 3 am arguments over whose turn it is to get up. Date nights? Yeah, right. Maybe if you count takeout on the couch while the baby sleeps.

But here's the deal: Your relationship matters, even more so now! So, how do you navigate this new normal and keep your connection strong? Here's your mission plan:

Tip 1: Teamwork Makes the Dream Work

Remember how you used to divvy up chores and stuff? That needs a major overhaul. Talk about how you can best support each other. Maybe you tackle night feeds while she catches up on sleep, or you take charge of laundry as she focuses on bonding time.

- **Communicate, communicate, communicate:** No, seriously. Even if it's a quick check-in while passing each other bottles, keep talking. What's frustrating you? What could make things a bit easier? Be open and honest.

Tip 2: Appreciation is Your Secret Weapon

It's easy to focus on what the other person *isn't* doing. Flip the script:

- **Verbalize the little things:** Thank her for getting the baby dressed and fed while you showered. It shows you notice and value her efforts.
- **Don't focus on the 'perfect':** She might not do things *exactly* how you would. A little flexibility goes a long way in those early months!

Tip 3: Carve Out Tiny 'Us' Moments

It won't be candlelit dinners at first, but you need

these sanity-savers.

- **5-minute coffee break:** Even just sitting together first thing in the morning can feel like a lifeline.
- **Tag team for personal time:** While one of you gives the baby a bath, the other gets 30 minutes for a walk, a book, or just some quiet. Trade off!
- **The 'No Baby Talk' rule:** For just 10 minutes a day, talk about something else! Your job, a funny show, anything to remind yourselves you're more than just parents.

Tip 4: When Romance Feels Impossible

Those first few months might not be overflowing with steamy vibes. That's okay! Focus on building intimacy in other ways.

- **Hugs and cuddles:** Simple physical affection matters when you're both exhausted.
- **Talk about your feelings:** Share hopes, fears, and just the funny moments of your new reality. That intimacy is just as powerful.
- **Don't put pressure on perfection:** 'Date night' could be ordering pizza and collapsing on the couch together. It's the 'together' part that counts.

The Bottom Line:

Your relationship will look different for a while. You'll both be going through major transitions.

But like every other aspect of being a dad, it's about patience, understanding, and adapting as you go. Remember, you're a team, and tackling this adventure together is the best gift you can give yourselves and your son.

PART 5: ADVANCED TACTICS FOR YEAR 1

19. SAFETY FIRST: BABYPROOFING YOUR HOME LIKE A PRO

Remember those carefree days when you didn't have to think about what dangers lurked behind every cabinet door? Those days are over, my friend! Once your little guy goes from sleepy newborn to mobile munchkin, your home becomes a giant obstacle course of potential hazards. But fear not, that's where babyproofing comes in!

Let's turn your normal pad into a fortress of safety. Here's how to go room-by-room, tackling the most common dangers:

The Living Room: HQ for Hazards

- **TV Time-Outs:** Secure your TV, whether it's mounted or on a stand. Curious climbers can't resist those big screens.
- **Coffee Table Combat:** Those sharp corners are headbump magnets. Cover them with bumpers or swap for a soft ottoman.
- **Outlet Overhaul:** Install outlet covers over EVERY outlet. Sure, they're a bit annoying, but

not nearly as annoying as a trip to the ER.

- **The Fireplace Fiasco:** Get a safety gate for your fireplace and keep lighters and matches out of reach.

The Kitchen: Cooking Up Caution

- **Cabinet Lockdown:** Use safety latches on drawers and cabinets with cleaning supplies, sharp knives, or anything breakable.
- **Stovetop Shield:** Install a stove guard to block curious hands from reaching those hot burners.
- **Beware the Oven:** Keep the oven door locked, even when not in use. Those little hands love to explore!

The Bathroom: Splash Zone Safety

- **Toilet Trouble:** Get a toilet lid lock. Babies are fascinated by water, and a toilet dip is not the kind of bath you want.
- **Medicine Mayhem:** Lock up all medications and vitamins in a high cabinet, out of reach and sight.
- **Slip 'N Slide Showdown:** Use non-slip mats in the tub and on the bathroom floor. Those wet surfaces get treacherous!

Additional Safety Tips

- **Down on Their Level:** Get down on your hands and knees and see the world from your baby's perspective. You'll spot all sorts of things you'd normally miss.

- **Window Watch:** Double-check window screens are secure and install window guards, especially on upper floors.
- **Blind Cord Chaos:** Blinds and curtains with dangling cords are strangulation hazards – remove them or use cord shorteners.
- **Think Small:** Check the floor for choking hazards – coins, batteries, small toys. Basically, if it can fit through a toilet paper roll, it's a danger.

Important Notes

- **Babyproof BEFORE they're mobile:** Don't wait until your little one's crawling to get safety conscious. Handle this way ahead of time!
- **Re-check Often:** As they grow and learn new skills, you'll need to constantly adapt and update your safety measures. What wasn't a problem yesterday could be a major issue tomorrow!

Remember, babyproofing doesn't mean your home has to look like a padded cell. It's about smart changes that reduce risks while still allowing your son the freedom to explore safely. And you know what? Even with the best babyproofing, accidents still happen. Be vigilant, forgive yourself when the inevitable bumps and scrapes occur, and never hesitate to call your pediatrician with any concerns.

Feeling like a safety superhero yet? Good! Tackling this babyproofing stuff gives you confidence and serious peace of mind.

20. OUT IN THE WORLD: TRAVEL, OUTINGS, AND CONQUERING ADVENTURES WITH YOUR LITTLE GUY

Remember those days when you could grab your backpack and head out on a whim? Well, those days might feel far away now, but that doesn't mean your adventurous spirit has to die with the arrival of your tiny travel companion.

Getting out and about with your baby opens up a whole new world of possibilities. Sure, it comes with extra planning and an insane amount of gear, but the rewards are worth it – I promise!

The Early Excursions

Let's be realistic – your first few trips will probably be short walks around the block or to the local coffee shop. And that's totally fine! Here's how to nail those mini-adventures:

- **The Gear Matters:** Get yourself a comfortable

baby carrier or stroller that works for your lifestyle. It makes a huge difference in how easily you can navigate the outside world.

- **Timing is Key:** Aim for outings after a nap and a good feed. A hangry, exhausted baby is not a happy travel companion.
- **Start small, build Big:** Build your confidence with neighborhood jaunts before planning an all-day adventure.

Tackling The Big Outings

Once you've got the basics down, time to level up those excursions. Here's what helps me when planning bigger adventures:

- **Packing List Master:** I keep a running packing list on my phone, so I don't forget those essentials like an extra outfit, wipes, and snacks (for baby and you!).
- **Embrace flexibility:** Babies thrive on routine, but they also roll with punches surprisingly well. Don't let a change in plans dampen your spirit.
- **Lower your expectations:** A visit to the zoo might mean seeing one animal and spending an hour in the gift shop. Guess what? That still counts as a win!

Adventure Ideas

Stuck on where to go? Here's some inspiration:

- **Nature Walks:** Parks, trails, even your

backyard are great for exploring with your little guy. Fresh air and new sights are a win-win.

- **Baby-Friendly Groups:** Look for local library story times, baby music classes, or playgroups. Meeting other parents can be a lifesaver.
- **Embrace the Tourist Spots:** Museums, aquariums, even a trip on a train can be super exciting through a baby's eyes.

The Dad Perspective

Getting out with your kid isn't just about entertaining him. It's great for you, too! It gets you outside of the house, forces you to try new things, and helps you build those dad-buds social connections.

And let's be honest, sometimes it's just nice to wear real pants and interact with actual adults, even for a little bit.

So yes, those adventures will look different than your pre-dad days. But trust me, they can be just as fulfilling, with the added bonus of sharing new experiences with your favorite little sidekick.

21. FOOD FIGHT! EXPANDING HIS PALATE, HANDLING PICKY EATING, AND MAKING MEALTIMES FUN

Okay, let's be honest – mealtimes with a baby can feel a bit like a scene from a food fight movie. There's pureed squash flying everywhere, yogurt somehow ends up in your hair, and that look of disgust on your son's face? Priceless.

But here's the thing: introducing your little one to new foods and developing healthy eating habits can be an enjoyable adventure rather than a daily struggle. Here's your mission plan for conquering those mealtime battles:

Mission Stage 1: Starting with Solids

Around the six-month mark, your little guy might be ready to start exploring the world of food beyond milk. Here's what you need to know:

- **Get the green light:** Check with your

pediatrician before starting solids. They'll help you assess his readiness and give guidance on safe first foods.

- **One at a time:** Introduce new foods slowly, waiting a few days between each one to check for allergies.
- **Texture is key:** Start with smooth purees, gradually progressing to thicker textures and soft, mashable foods.

Mission Stage 2: Embracing the Mess

Babies learn by exploring, and mealtimes are no exception. Yes, it will get messy!

- **Protect your battle zone:** Invest in a good splat mat, bibs with catch-all pockets, and washable clothes for you both. Embrace the chaos!
- **Let him get hands-on:** Put some food directly on his tray and let him explore the textures, smells, and yes, even flinging bits around is part of the learning process.
- **Make those funny faces:** Be a little goofy! Exaggerated expressions (surprise, disgust, utter delight) encourage him to try new things.

Mission Stage 3: Defeating the Picky Eater

Don't panic when that first adorable open-mouthed enthusiasm for food morphs into a stubborn refusal to eat anything green. Picky eating is entirely normal!

- **Keep offering, no pressure**: It can take multiple tries for babies to accept new foods. Simply offer a variety without forcing him to eat.
- **Get creative**: Cut food into fun shapes, offer colorful veggie sticks with dip, or even try the old 'airplane spoon' trick.
- **Don't be a short-order cook**: Avoid making separate meals for your picky eater. Offer healthy options, and let him choose what (and how much) he eats. He won't starve himself!

Bonus Mission: Making it Fun

Mealtimes can be a fantastic time to bond and encourage development. Here's how:

- **Eat together**: As much as possible, have family meals and let him see you enjoying the same foods. Monkey see, monkey do!
- **Tell food stories**: Talk about where food comes from, make shopping trips an adventure by picking out colorful produce, maybe even grow a simple herb in a pot.
- **Playtime at the table**: Sing silly songs about food, make up stories about the broccoli 'trees', let him play with (washable) spoons and dishes while you eat.

Remember, you're not just feeding his body; you're shaping his relationship with food. Keep it positive, be patient, and don't forget to have fun. Before you know it, you might have a little foodie on your hands!

22. TAMING THE TANTRUMS: UNDERSTANDING MELTDOWNS AND HOW TO KEEP YOUR COOL

Remember the days when your biggest worry was a diaper blowout? Adorable, right? Well, get ready, because as your little guy grows, we're entering a new world of emotions. Welcome to the wild and wonderful phase of tantrums!

The first time my son had a full-blown meltdown in the middle of the grocery store, I felt like everyone was judging my parenting skills. Sweat was forming, my face was turning red... yep, I was on the verge of my own tantrum. But here's the thing: tantrums are a totally normal part of toddler development.

Why the Drama, Little Guy?

Think of it this way: Your son's brain is developing

at lightning speed, but his communication skills are still lagging behind. Sometimes, big emotions build up and the only way he knows how to express them is through a noisy, chaotic explosion – a.k.a., a tantrum.

Common tantrum triggers include:

- **Frustration:** He wants to do something himself but doesn't have the skills yet.
- **Overwhelm:** Too much noise, stimulation, or new situations.
- **Communication struggles:** He can't find the words to express how he feels.
- **Hunger/Tiredness:** Hey, we all get cranky when these basic needs aren't met!

Keeping Your Cool (Seriously, How?)

When the meltdown hits, it's easy to feel helpless or even angry. Here are some strategies:

1. **Take a deep breath (or ten):** Reacting in the heat of the moment will only escalate things.
2. **Safety first:** Make sure he's not going to hurt himself or others. If you're in a public place, find a quieter spot if possible.
3. **Empathize, don't dismiss:** "You seem really mad that we have to leave the park" shows him you understand, even if you can't give in to his demands.
4. **Offer limited choices:** "Do you want your

blue cup or your red cup?" gives him a sense of control within boundaries.

5. **Distraction sometimes works:** With younger toddlers, switching gears ("Look at the airplane!") can redirect their attention.

6. **When it's over, connect:** Once he's calmed down, a hug and a simple "That was a big feeling, wasn't it?" helps him feel safe and understood.

Important Reminders:

- **Tantrums aren't intentional misbehavior:** He's not doing it to be manipulative; he's genuinely overwhelmed.

- **Don't give in to avoid the scene:** Giving him what he wants during a tantrum will only reinforce the behavior.

- **Sometimes, you just gotta ride it out:** Stay calm, stay safe, and remind yourself *this too shall pass*.

- **You're not a failure:** Every parent of a toddler has been there. You're doing the best you can!

Preventing Future Meltdowns (Is It Even Possible?)

You can't eliminate tantrums entirely, but you can reduce them:

- **Routines rock:** Predictable schedules for meals and sleep help him feel secure.

- **Warnings help:** Give him notice before transitions ("Five more minutes at the playground, then it's time to go!").
- **Head off hanger:** Always have snacks on hand!

Tantrums are a tough part of parenting, but they're a sign that your child is growing. With patience, understanding, and (most importantly) a sense of humor, you'll weather this stormy phase and come out stronger on the other side.

23. DISCIPLINE BEGINS: SETTING POSITIVE BOUNDARIES AND GENTLE GUIDANCE

Okay, let's talk about a word that might strike fear into the heart of any new dad: Discipline. Before your little guy is even walking, you're probably already picturing years of timeouts and yelling matches. Take a deep breath. Here's the thing: discipline with a baby isn't about punishment; it's about setting the foundation for good behavior, safety, and strong bonds

Start with Love and Understanding

Remember, your baby isn't intentionally trying to make your life difficult (yet!). He's exploring the world, figuring out how things work. Sometimes that means pulling your hair, dumping out his food, or flinging the cat's water bowl across the room. Instead of anger, try curiosity: What is he trying to understand by doing that?

Here are some key things to keep in mind:

- **Tiny brains understand less**: They can't reason the way we do, so explaining why something's wrong won't get you far.
- **Redirection is your friend**: When he's doing something unsafe or undesirable, distract and replace! Offer a different, safe toy, or change the environment.
- **Consistency matters**: If something's off-limits one day but okay the next, he'll be confused. Do your best to have clear and consistent "house rules".

Setting Gentle Boundaries

As your little explorer gets more mobile, boundaries are no longer an option, they're a safety necessity! Here's how to handle those "no" moments effectively while still being a loving, responsive dad:

Keep it simple and calm: Just say "No", firmly, with eye contact. A drawn-out explanation isn't going to sink in with a baby.

- **Consistency is Key**: Use the same tone and simple language every time the behavior happens. He might not understand the word yet, but he'll start to associate it with being stopped.
- **No Yelling**: Shouting only ramps up everyone's stress levels. A firm, calm "no"

carries more weight.

- **Body Language Matters:** Your disapproving frown and direct eye contact reinforce the message.

Immediately remove him from the situation: Pick him up and move him away from that enticing electrical socket.

- **Action > Words:** Don't get into a power struggle with your little guy. Simply remove him from the situation and redirect his attention.
- **Make the "Bad Thing" Unavailable:** If possible, block off forbidden areas or put tempting objects out of sight to set him up for success.

Offer a positive alternative: Give him something safe and more interesting to play with.

- **The Art of Distraction:** Redirection is your best friend! A fun toy can instantly switch his focus from something he shouldn't be touching.
- **Choice Works Wonders:** Instead of a straight "no", try offering two acceptable options. "Do you want the ball or the blocks?" gives him a sense of control within safe boundaries.

Praise the good stuff!: When he's playing nicely on his own, acknowledge it! "Wow, I love how you're building with the blocks!" reinforces the

behaviors you DO want to see.

- **The Power of the Positive:** Babies thrive on praise and attention. Highlight the good behaviors, and those are the ones he'll be motivated to repeat.
- **Specific Praise:** Don't just say "good boy!" Label the specific behavior you like: "Good job staying on your blanket!" This helps him associate the praise with the action.

Remember:

- **Don't Expect Perfection:** Boundary testing is how he learns. Stay patient and consistent, and he'll gradually get the hang of it.
- **It's a Process:** As he gets older, you CAN start giving brief explanations alongside your "no." ("We don't touch the stove because it's hot!")
- **Pick Your Battles:** Prioritize safety. Sometimes it's okay to let him explore a mess if it's harmless, so you save your "nos" for the truly important things.

Dealing with Meltdowns

Even the most adorable baby can unleash a full-blown meltdown! The key is understanding meltdowns aren't about being 'bad'. They're a sign of big emotions your little one doesn't know how to handle yet. Here's how you can navigate those stormy seas:

Stay calm yourself: Easier said than done, I know! But getting upset will escalate things.

- **Take a Dad Timeout:** If you feel yourself about to lose it, hand the baby off to your partner if possible, or put him in a safe place (like the crib) and take a few minutes to compose yourself.

- **Deep Breaths are Your Weapon:** Simple but effective. A few deep breaths help reset your nervous system and bring you back to rational-dad mode.

- **It's Not Personal:** Remember, his meltdown is about him struggling with big emotions, not about you being a bad dad.

Validate the feelings: "I know you're angry!" You don't have to give in, but showing empathy helps him feel understood.

- **Name the Emotion:** Labeling what he's feeling helps him learn to identify his emotions in the future. Say things like, "You seem really frustrated!" or "You're so mad right now!".

- **Empathy, Not Approval:** You're not saying his behavior is okay, but you're acknowledging the struggle he's going through. This goes a long way in calming the storm.

- **No Shaming:** Avoid phrases like "Stop crying!" or "You're being a bad boy!". This only makes him feel worse about an already overwhelming situation.

Wait it out if safe: Sometimes they just need to release that big feeling. If he's in a safe place, let the storm pass, being nearby for comfort once he's calmed down.

- **Safe Space:** Make sure he's not in danger of hurting himself or others. Sometimes removing him from the situation to a quiet space can help, but sometimes the meltdown has to run its course.
- **Your Calm Presence:** You might need to just sit there and weather the storm. It's hard to see your little one so upset, but your presence is reassuring, even if he's pushing you away right now.
- **Afterwards:** Once he's past the worst of it, offer comfort with gentle words and cuddles. There's no need for a big lecture – just move on and reconnect.

Important to Remember:

- **Brain Development:** His brain is still immature, and he literally doesn't have the skills to regulate his emotions yet. That's where you come in!
- **Every Kid is Different:** Some babies are more intense than others. Don't compare your little one to other kids – focus on understanding and meeting his needs.
- **It Gets Easier (I Swear!):** As he grows and

you get better at reading his cues, meltdowns become easier to manage, and sometimes even prevent altogether.

Remember: It's a Learning Process

Don't expect perfection – from your son or from yourself! Some days you'll have it together, and some days the yelling will happen because you're only human. The most important thing is:

- **Model the behavior you want:** How you handle frustration, anger, and saying "no" is what he's really absorbing.
- **It's about connection, not control:** Discipline isn't a power struggle. It's about teaching, guiding, and keeping that bond with your little guy strong. You're on the same team!

24. PLAYTIME POWER-UPS: ACTIVITIES THAT BOOST HIS DEVELOPMENT AND YOUR BOND

Okay, enough with the diapers and sleep schedules for a minute (although I know we'll be right back to those soon!). Let's talk about the fun stuff — playing with your little guy! Playtime isn't just about having a good time; it's like rocket fuel for his development. Plus, it's the perfect way to strengthen your bond and start creating amazing memories together.

Here's the thing: You don't need fancy toys or complicated activities. The best playtime sessions are simple, follow his lead, and focus on connecting with each other.

Age-by-Age Playtime Power-Ups

Let's break down some ideas tailored to different ages and stages:

Newborn To 3 Months:

Tummy Time Adventures: A few minutes on his tummy (while supervised!) strengthens neck muscles and is way more exciting than it sounds. Add a colorful toy in front of him for motivation.

- **Why It Matters:** Tummy time is your little guy's first workout! It helps him build strength for rolling over, crawling, and avoiding the dreaded "flat head".
- **Make It Fun:**
  - Get on his level! Lie on the floor facing him to make it more engaging.
  - Sing silly songs or make funny noises to encourage him to look up.
  - Place a rolled-up towel under his chest for slight support, making it easier to lift up.
  - Dangle a high-contrast toy or mirror just above his eye line.

Sensory Stimulation: Soft fabrics, gentle sounds, contrasting black and white images – engage his developing senses!

- **His Amazing Senses:** His vision is still blurry and he's drawn to strong contrasts and repetitive sounds. This is a prime time to engage those developing senses safely.
- **Ways to Play:**
  - Offer different textures: A soft blanket,

a crinkly toy, even your own skin! Let his little hands explore.

o   Talk to him throughout the day: He's soaking up the sound of your voice – narrate everything, even the mundane stuff!

o   Hold black and white patterned images a few inches from his face: They're surprisingly captivating to newborns.

o   Music Time: Introduce soft lullabies, nature sounds, or even simple melodies you make up.

Face Time: Get close, smile, make silly faces, and talk to him in a high-pitched voice. This simple interaction is HUGE for his brain development.

- **Bonding Power:** Your face is the best toy! The more expressions, silly voices, and sweet words he sees and hears, the stronger his neural connections grow.
- **Dad Tip:**
  o   Exaggerate your facial expressions: Wide eyes, big smiles, sticking out your tongue – he'll love the novelty.
  o   Don't be afraid of high-pitched "baby talk": It's naturally engaging to little ones and highlights different tones in your voice.
  o   Time it right: Connect when he's alert and not fussy, so the experience is more positive for both of you.

- o   Respond to his cues: If he seems overwhelmed, take a break! Even short bursts of interaction are beneficial.

4-6 Months:

Reach and Grasp: Introduce rattles, crinkly toys, and anything he can easily grab. This works those hand muscles for some awesome future block-building skills.

- **Variety is Key:** Offer toys with different shapes, sizes, and textures. This helps refine his grasp and keeps playtime interesting.
- **The Household Explorer:** Safe household objects (wooden spoon, plastic bowl, etc.) are just as fascinating as expensive toys.
- Play "Drop It" (On Purpose!): Let him intentionally drop toys from his high chair or play mat. He's learning about cause and effect – plus it's hilarious.
- **Two is Better Than One:** Encourage passing toys from hand to hand – this strengthens coordination.

Sing-Along Time: Bust out those nursery rhymes, invent silly songs with his name – doesn't matter if you're off-key, he loves the sound of your voice.

- **Music Maestro:** Shake rattles along to the beat, or tap out rhythms on pots and pans. He's soaking up the musical patterns.
- **Dance Party with Dad:** Hold him and sway to music. Exposing him to rhythm and movement is great for coordination.

- **Repetition is His Jam:** Don't worry about getting bored singing the same song over and over. That repetition is how he learns!
- **The Soundtrack of Life:** Sing while changing him, during bathtime...anytime! It makes daily routines more fun and builds language skills.

The Floor is Lava!: Put him on a blanket and gently pull him around the room for a new perspective. Giggles guaranteed.

- **Sightseeing Tour:** Point out interesting things as you pull him along – the ceiling fan, his reflection in a mirror, the dog asleep on the rug.
- **Core Strength Workout:** This movement encourages him to engage those core muscles as he tries to balance.
- **Safety First:** Stay on a soft surface, go slow at first, and be aware of objects he might grab as you pass (cords, dangling houseplants, etc.).
- **Narrate The Adventure:** Talk about what you're doing as you go ("Whee! Let's go see the kitchen!")

7-9 Months:

Obstacle Course Champion: Pillows, blankets, even you become challenges as he starts crawling. Cheer him on as he conquers each new hurdle.

- Mobility Milestone: Crawling is a big deal! He's figuring out how to control his body in a whole new way, and getting stronger every day.
- Dad's Role:
    - Enthusiastic Sportscaster: Narrate his progress in a playful way ("Ooh, he's going under the chair! Can he make it out the other side?").
    - Obstacle Course Creator: Arrange soft cushions, rolled-up blankets, and tunnels for him to navigate. (Bonus points if you crawl right alongside him!)
    - Safety Spotter: Be close by to rearrange anything that could become a tipping hazard.

Peek-a-Boo Master: This classic game never gets old. It teaches object permanence (things still exist even when he can't see them) and is just plain fun.

- Cognitive Development Boost: Peek-a-boo helps him grasp that you continue to exist even when you disappear – a surprisingly complex concept!

- Dad's Role:
  - Go Big or Go Home: Exaggerated expressions, hiding behind absurd objects, and popping out with a big "Boo!" add to the excitement.
  - Wait for It: Extend the pause before you reappear, building anticipation. The longer the wait, the bigger the giggle-filled reaction!
  - Variation is Key: Hide yourself, hide a favorite toy – the change-up keeps things interesting.

Exploration Station: Open safe drawers and cabinets low to the ground. Let him pull out pots, pans, wooden spoons...supervised kitchen chaos is his new favorite activity.

- Sensory Playground: Your kitchen contains a treasure trove of interesting textures, sounds, and shapes. Let him loose (under close supervision!) to explore.
- Dad's Role:
  - Safety Prep: Designate a baby-safe cabinet or drawer, filled with unbreakable, non-choking items. Think plastic bowls, wooden spoons, measuring cups, etc.
  - The Narrator: Describe what he's holding and the sounds he's making ("That's a shiny pan! Bang, bang, bang!").
  - Don't Expect Tidiness: Embrace the joyful

mess! Focus on the fun of discovery, not on keeping the kitchen spotless.

10-12 Months:

Ballin' Out: Rolling a ball back and forth might seem basic, but it works on coordination and social skills. Add in goofy sound effects for extra fun.

- **Beyond the Basics:** Rolling a ball develops hand-eye coordination, teaches cause and effect (he kicks, the ball moves), and is the foundation for future ball skills!
- **Dad Upgrade:**
  - Start close, then gradually increase the distance for a challenge.
  - Make silly whooshing sounds as the ball rolls, then encourage him to imitate you.
  - Introduce different textures: Try a soft ball, a bumpy ball, a bouncy ball – all are interesting to explore.
  - Get Competitive (kind of): "Block" his roll and then let him triumphantly push through, building confidence and giggles.

Let's Get Stacked: Big, soft blocks are perfect for building towers and knocking them down with glee.

- **Master Builder:** Stacking blocks builds fine motor skills, problem-solving, and introduces basic engineering ("Why did it fall?"). Destruction is equally valuable!

- **Dad Upgrade:**
  - "Help" him build a tower, then celebrate its epic destruction!
  - Use blocks for peek-a-boo: Hide under a blanket-covered stack and surprise him.
  - Make it a sorting game: Put different shaped blocks into a bucket, encouraging him to find the matching hole.
  - Talk about colors and shapes: "You found the big blue block!"

Story Time Snuggles: Board books with bright pictures are great now. Point out objects, describe colors, and let him turn the pages.

- **Bookworm Beginnings:** This sets the stage for a lifelong love of reading. Comforting snuggles + books = happy brain connections.
- **Dad Upgrade:**
  - Animal noises over words: Point at a picture of a cat and instead of reading "cat", let out a dramatic "MEEEOOWWW!"
  - Let him lead: Follow his interest as he points at pages, even if it's out of order.
  - Make it interactive: Ask "Where's the doggy?" and help him find it.
  - Chew-proof books are best: Babies experience the world through their mouth, so invest in sturdy, chew-safe books!

Remember, the BEST playtime is:

- **Responsive:** Watch his cues. Is he interested, overwhelmed, or getting tired? Adjust as needed. Short and sweet sessions are often better than marathon playtimes.
- **Silly:** Don't be afraid to let loose with your inner goofball. Exaggerated expressions, funny sounds, and playful tickles spark those delightful belly laughs.
- **Gadget-Free:** Put away your phone and give him your full attention. He'll notice and appreciate the one-on-one connection.

Playtime is about more than toys or hitting milestones. It's about building the foundation for a strong, loving relationship that will last a lifetime. So, let go of any pressure to "do it right," get on the floor, and discover the joy of playtime with your little man!

25. SPECIAL AGENT TRAINING: HANDLING HOLIDAYS, FAMILY GATHERINGS, AND BIG EVENTS

Alright Dad, time to upgrade your mission. You've mastered the basics of feeding and diapering on home turf, but now it's time to take your little agent out into the wider world. Big family gatherings, holidays, and those first special events can feel like a whole new level of chaos, but no worries – we'll strategize and make sure you're prepared.

Mission Objective: Keep Calm and Parent On

Whether it's Grandma's famous Thanksgiving feast or your little guy's first birthday party, these events add a whole new layer of parenting logistics. The goal is to make it through while keeping your baby happy (as much as possible) and maintaining your own sanity.

The Briefing: What to Expect

- **Sensory overload:** Babies get overwhelmed easily. All the noises, faces, and new smells at big events can lead to meltdowns and fussy spells.
- **Schedule disruptions:** Even if you're an expert at naptime at home, don't expect things to magically stick to the schedule when you're out.
- **Unwanted 'advice':** Be prepared for everyone, from well-meaning aunts to complete strangers, to have strong opinions about how you're doing things.

Your Agent Toolkit

- **Pack like a pro:** Bring way more supplies than you think you'll need. Diaper changes on the go, a spare outfit (or two), his favorite soothing toy – it's better to overpack than get caught unprepared.
- **Find quiet spaces:** Locate a designated 'chill out' zone beforehand, whether it's an empty bedroom or a quiet spot outside. This is where you can retreat with your baby for feeding, calming meltdowns, or a quick break.
- **Practice saying "no":** You'll encounter folks who want to hold the baby even if he's crying, or offer him foods he shouldn't be eating yet. Be polite but firm in setting boundaries to

protect him.

- **Adjust your expectations:** It's okay if your baby sleeps through the entire holiday dinner or cries through photos. Focus on enjoying the moments you CAN, not forcing things to be picture-perfect.

Holiday-Specific Strategies

- **Thanksgiving:** Be prepared for people trying to sneak a taste of mashed potatoes to your baby! (Not cool, Grandma.) Talk to family beforehand about your feeding plan.
- **Christmas/Hanukkah etc.:** Don't feel pressured to buy a ton of presents. One or two simple, age-appropriate toys are plenty. Overwhelm is real with babies!
- **Birthdays:** Your baby might be more interested in the wrapping paper than the actual gifts – totally normal! Keep things simple and focus on enjoying the moment.

Remember, It's Your Mission

Don't feel like you have to say 'yes' to every event or tradition. If something sounds too overwhelming, it's okay to set boundaries. If you need to leave early, do it! Protecting your little guy's needs and your own peace of mind is the most important part of the mission.

Above all, try to have some fun amidst the chaos. Seeing those big events through your baby's eyes adds a whole new layer of magic. And hey, all that strategizing and adaptability? That's some expert-level dad training right there!

PART 6: THE SUPER DAD LEGACY

26. MISSION ACCOMPLISHED? NOPE! THE SUPERHERO JOURNEY CONTINUES

Okay, high five! You survived the first year of fatherhood – the sleepless nights, the diaper disasters, the mysterious crying jags. You, my friend, are a seasoned dad veteran now. Give yourself a serious pat on the back, then pour yourself a strong cup of coffee. Because guess what? The adventure has just begun!

Your tiny baby is now a walking, talking (sort of), tantrum-throwing (maybe) toddler on a whole new level of exploration. This next chapter of the dad journey is filled with wonder, laughter, and probably a few more gray hairs. Let's get you ready:

- **Toddler-proofing Your World: The Next Stage of Safety and Independence** Safety was important with a baby, but it's a whole new ballgame with a toddler. They're faster, more curious, and determined to get into everything. We'll cover how to turn your home into a safe haven for a little explorer.

- **Discipline with Love: Setting Gentle Boundaries and Positive Guidance** As your little one tests those limits (and trust me, they will), it's time to start setting some loving boundaries. This isn't about punishment, but teaching him right from wrong in a way that supports his development.

- **Tech and Your Tot: Managing Screen Time Responsibly** Love them or hate them, screens are part of the world now. We'll navigate how to handle screen time for toddlers, finding the balance between letting them explore technology and protecting their developing brains.

- **Family Traditions: Creating Special Moments that Last a Lifetime** Whether it's big holidays or silly made-up rituals, traditions are the glue that holds families together. We'll brainstorm fun ways to make unique memories and pass on traditions to your little guy.

- **The Road Ahead: Ongoing Joys and Challenges of Being a Dad** Being a dad is a lifelong journey, constantly changing and evolving. We'll take a moment to look ahead and embrace both the amazing times to come and those inevitable bumps in the road.

You've Got This, Dad: Reflections on Year One and Celebrating Your Journey

Before we dive into toddlerhood, take a breath. Think about how far you've come. Look back at that wide-eyed new dad holding a tiny baby, and now see the confident father you've become.

You've learned, you've messed up, you've laughed, and you've loved this kid with everything you've got. The superhero costume might be a bit worn around the edges, but your superpowers are stronger than ever. Cheers to you, dad!

27. TODDLER-PROOFING YOUR WORLD: THE NEXT STAGE OF SAFETY AND INDEPENDENCE

Remember a few months ago when your biggest worry was figuring out how to change a diaper? Well, prepare yourself – things are about to get a whole lot more... mobile. Once your little guy figures out how to crawl, walk, and climb, your once familiar home turns into a brand new obstacle course – one littered with potential hazards.

But fear not, dads! This chapter is your guide to turning your house into a toddler-friendly zone, creating a balance between safety and those awesome bursts of newly gained independence.

Step 1: Get Down On Their Level

The best way to spot dangers is to literally see the world from your toddler's perspective. Get down on your hands and knees and crawl around, paying close attention to things he might find particularly interesting. Here's what to watch out for:

- **Dangerous Temptations:** Electrical outlets, cleaning supplies, medicine bottles – anything small, brightly colored, or within reach is a potential choking hazard or source of accidental poisoning.
- **Climbing Adventures:** Stairs, chairs, windows, and furniture are no longer just objects, they're invitations for daredevil exploration.
- **Household Weaponry:** Sharp corners on tables, heavy objects that can topple over, even those adorable houseplants (many are toxic if nibbled).

Step 2: The Lock-It-Down Lockdown

Now, it's not about making your home look like a padded cell, but smart modifications are key. Here's your starter checklist:

- **Outlet covers:** They're cheap and easy – use them EVERYWHERE.
- **Cabinet locks:** Go for magnetic or hidden latches, those flimsy plastic ones are no match for a curious toddler. Focus on low cabinets and those containing cleaning supplies and other dangers.
- **Toilet locks:** If you haven't gotten these yet, do it now. Toddlers are fascinated by water, and toilets are extra tempting.
- **Door knob covers:** Prevent your little Houdini from escaping his room for a 3 am adventure (or locking you in the bathroom).
- **Gates and guards:** Essential for stairs (top and bottom!), fireplaces, and any 'no-go' zones in your house.
- **Furniture anchors:** Secure those bookcases, dressers, and even TVs to the wall. Toddlers love to climb, and you don't want anything tipping over.

Step 3: Out Of Sight, Out Of Reach

Sometimes, the best defense is a strategic retreat. Do a sweep of your house and make these changes:

- **Poison control:** Move cleaning supplies, medications, and anything potentially toxic to high shelves or locked cabinets. Your kitchen and bathroom are high-risk zones.
- **Choking Hazards:** Coins, batteries, small toys, and anything that can fit in a toddler's mouth need to be relocated. Get vigilant about picking up stuff off the floor.
- **The Blind Spot:** Cords from blinds and curtains are a strangulation hazard. Secure them out of reach or consider cordless options.
- **Kitchen Dangers:** Use stove knob covers and install a guard around the stove, if possible. Consider moving knives, sharp utensils, and heavy pots and pans.

Bonus Tip: Create a "Yes" Space

Toddlerhood is all about exploration. It's unfair (and frankly impossible!) to make your entire house off-limits. Designate a room or area that's safe for him to roam freely. Fill it with age-appropriate toys, books, and comfy furniture he can climb on and off without worrying you.

Step 4: Constant Vigilance (But Don't Drive Yourself Nuts)

Even with the best toddler-proofing, accidents can still happen. Here's how to strike that balance between safety and freedom:

- **Supervise, but don't hover:** Be present without micromanaging his every move. You want him to learn and explore, just under your watchful eye.
- **Explain the "why":** Even though they're tiny, start having simple talks about safety. "The stove is hot, ouch!" "We keep medicine up high so it doesn't make you sick." They'll start to understand.
- **Redirect, redirect, redirect:** If he's constantly drawn to something dangerous, distract him with an enticing alternative. It'll save your sanity (and his safety).
- **Learn infant/child first aid:** Empower yourself with essential knowledge just in case.

28. DISCIPLINE WITH LOVE: SETTING GENTLE BOUNDARIES AND POSITIVE GUIDANCE

Remember when you thought changing diapers would be the hardest part of being a dad? Well, welcome to the world of toddler tantrums, hurled food, and those defiant "NO!" screams! It's enough to make any dad want to hide under the couch.

But hey, this is also where the real magic of parenting starts to happen. This is when you get to guide your little guy, teaching him about rules, self-control, and ultimately helping him become a responsible, kind human being. The goal isn't about being a drill sergeant; it's about setting up your child for success by combining clear boundaries with a whole lot of love.

Why Bother With Discipline? (Besides the Obvious Meltdown Prevention)

- **Safety First:** Little kids naturally lack impulse control. Teaching them about what's safe and what's off-limits can literally be a lifesaver.

- **Respecting Others:** Understanding boundaries helps kids learn empathy and how to treat others with kindness.
- **Building Confidence:** Believe it or not, clear rules and routines give kids a sense of security and predictability, which actually lowers anxiety, not raises it.

Okay, But How Do I Do It Without Losing My Mind?

First of all, ditch the idea of "perfect" discipline. Toddlers are a work in progress (and honestly, so are we as dads!). Here's a better mindset to aim for:

- **Be Proactive, Not Just Reactive:** Set up routines and clear expectations for common situations (bedtime, mealtime, getting dressed) to head off meltdowns before they start.
- **Focus on Connection:** Discipline works best when you have a strong bond with your child. Spend one-on-one time playing and just being present each day.
- **See the World Through Their Eyes:** Toddlers aren't being defiant on purpose. They're still learning how to handle big emotions, wants, and frustrations.

Practical Strategies for Positive Discipline

- **Start with "Yes":** Instead of always saying "no," find ways to say "yes" safely. Instead of

"No running with the scissors!" try "Scissors are for cutting paper at the table, let's go find some!"

- **Set Clear Rules:** Keep them simple and age-appropriate. Instead of a vague "Be nice," you might have a rule like, "Gentle hands on our friends."
- **Consequences Over Punishment:** Focus on natural or logical consequences. If toys get thrown, they go away for a while. This teaches more effectively than yelling or timeouts.
- **Offer Choices (Within Limits):** Give your child a sense of control: "Do you want the blue shirt or the red shirt?". This decreases power struggles.
- **Praise the Good Stuff:** Catch them being kind, following a rule, or trying to calm themselves down. Positive attention is way more powerful than focusing on negatives.

When Meltdowns DO Happen (and They Will!)

- **Stay Calm (Easier Said Than Done, I Know):** Take a deep breath before reacting. If you're losing it, your kid will too. It's okay to walk away for a minute to regroup.
- **Acknowledge the Feelings:** Say things like, "I see you're really mad you can't play outside right now. It's okay to feel mad." This helps them learn to name their emotions.
- **Offer Comfort When Ready:** Once the storm passes, offer a hug or some soothing words.

Talk about why they were upset and how to handle it differently next time.

What About Timeouts?

Timeouts can be a controversial topic. Some experts use them effectively, but often they're misused, becoming more about punishment than teaching. If you do use timeouts, here's the twist:

- **"Timeout" = Time IN:** Instead of sending them away, have a special 'calm down' spot with pillows and a favorite book. Let them come to you when they're ready to talk.
- **Short and Sweet:** One minute per year of age is a good rule of thumb. Long timeouts do more harm than good.
- **The Talk is Key:** After the timeout, focus on repairing the connection. Talk about what happened and discuss better choices for the future.

29. TECH AND YOUR TOT: MANAGING SCREEN TIME RESPONSIBLY

Okay, let's tackle a big one: screen time. As dads, most of us grew up with technology, but raising a kid in the age of smartphones, tablets, and nonstop kids' YouTube channels is a whole new ball game. It seems like everyone has an opinion on what's okay and what's not, which adds another layer of worry to parenthood.

But here's the thing: while screens can be overwhelming, they're not all evil. It's about finding a balance that works for your family and sets your son up for success in this digital world.

The Basics: What Do the Experts Say?

The American Academy of Pediatrics has some pretty clear guidelines on screen time for those under two years old:

- **Under 18 months:** They recommend avoiding screens altogether, with the exception of video chatting with family and friends.

- **18 months to 2 years**: Very limited screen time, with a parent co-viewing to help them understand what they're seeing. Choose high-quality educational content above shows with no substance.

Why so strict? Because the little brain is developing at an insane pace during those first two years. Too much screen time can interfere with face-to-face interactions, physical play, and those crucial language-learning opportunities that happen through conversation.

But...It's Real Life

I get it, as a parent myself, sometimes you just need five minutes to finish a meal, answer an email, whatever! A short burst of kid-friendly screen time to save your sanity is not the end of the world. The key is moderation and always prioritizing those real-world interactions.

Here's a breakdown of how I try to approach screens:

The First Year: Low-Tech Zone

For the most part, we tried to keep our son's world screen-free during his first year. There were occasional family video calls and sometimes I'd sneak in a quick glance at my phone while he played, but it wasn't a regular occurrence. Instead, we focused on tons of reading, singing, and hands-on sensory play.

From One to Two: Limited Introduction

Once he hit the toddler stage, we started gradually introducing little bits of screen time. There's a great app called 'Khan Academy Kids' with interactive games and learning activities we used for short stretches when we really needed it. We always sat with him, talked about what he was seeing, and made sure it was a positive experience.

Now: Balance is Key

Now that he's older, we still try to keep screens as an occasional 'treat', not an everyday habit. There are days when he watches a short episode of "Daniel Tiger" while I cook dinner, and sometimes if we're on a long car ride, a tablet helps pass the time. But we also have plenty of screen-free days, especially when the weather's nice and we can play outside.

Making Your Own Screen Smart Rules

Every family needs to find the approach that works for them. Here are some questions to guide your thinking:

- **Set screen time limits:** How much is too much? Will you have certain times of day that are screen-free zones?
- **Content is king:** What will you allow your child to watch? Educational shows and apps over mindless YouTube binges.

- **Co-viewing is crucial:** Especially in the beginning, watch with him, talk about the characters and stories. Make it an active experience, not passive zoning out.
- **Screens don't replace real-world play:** No matter how amazing the app is, it'll never replace building blocks, running around, and getting messy.
- **Model good tech habits:** If you're always glued to your phone, it sends a mixed message about screen time rules.

Beyond Strict Limits: Creating a Tech-Healthy Kid

The goal isn't just about limiting screens. It's about raising a kid with a healthy relationship with technology. Here are some additional things to keep in mind as your son gets older:

- **Be aware of online safety:** As he gains access to the internet, talking about safe browsing, not sharing personal information, and being kind online will become essential conversations.
- **Encourage creativity over consumption:** Look for apps and games that let him create art, build things, and solve problems – not just passively watch content.
- **Prioritize real life experiences:** Make sure outdoor time, reading books, and hands-on activities always remain a huge part of his

childhood.

- **Tech breaks are important:** Help him learn to step away from a screen and relax without needing that constant stimulation.

30. FAMILY TRADITIONS: CREATING SPECIAL MOMENTS THAT LAST A LIFETIME

Remember that feeling when you were a kid, and your birthday seemed like the biggest, best day of the year? Or how excited you'd get for family holidays? It wasn't just the presents or the food (though those were awesome); it was that sense of something...special. That's what traditions are all about!

As dads, we have this amazing chance to create those magical experiences for our kids. Think of traditions as the glue that holds families together. They add rhythm and predictability to our lives, give kids something to look forward to, and create lasting memories.

Now, here's the thing about tradition – it doesn't have to be fancy or complicated. Even the smallest things, done consistently, become meaningful over time.

Let's explore why family traditions rock, and then I'll share some fun ideas to get you started!

The Power of Tradition

- **A sense of belonging**: Traditions remind kids they're part of something bigger than themselves, creating a sense of identity and security.

- **Reduces stress**: Knowing what to expect, especially for little ones, can help them feel more settled during times of change or big transitions.

- **Strengthens bonds**: Shared experiences and inside jokes from those silly traditions create powerful connections that last a lifetime.

- **Teaches values**: Whether it's a holiday tradition focused on giving back or a weekly family game night, these rituals reinforce what's important to your family.

- **Pure and simple FUN**: Life with a baby is full of routine. Traditions are your chance to shake things up and add in a dash of joy!

Okay, but where to start?

Think about these when brainstorming:

- **Your own childhood**: Were there any traditions you loved? Maybe a special pancake breakfast on Saturdays or building blanket forts on rainy days? Now's your chance to pass them on!

- **Interests and hobbies:** If your family loves the outdoors, start a tradition of a yearly camping trip. Bookworms? Make Friday nights 'library night'. Build traditions around things you already enjoy.
- **Holidays both big and small:** The obvious ones are great, but think about celebrating even minor holidays (like National Talk Like a Pirate Day – seriously, get those costumes ready!)
- **Everyday rituals:** Bedtime stories, a special way to say good morning, or a designated 'family walk' time can become cherished traditions.

Let's Get Creative - Tradition Ideas for Every Stage

- **Baby & Toddler Traditions:**
  - A special bathtime song you always sing
  - Taking monthly photos at the same spot to see them grow
  - "First food Friday" where they try a new food each week
  - A yearly handprint ornament for the holidays
- **Preschooler & Up:**
  - Build a birthday "time capsule" where they write a letter to their future self
  - Choose a special place to visit every year (park, zoo, beach)
  - Have them help bake a "family recipe"

> each holiday season
> o Volunteer together for a cause you all care about

Tips for Success

- **Be consistent:** The more regular the tradition, the more meaningful it becomes.
- **Make it interactive:** Let your child have a say in the activities or help with the setup – it increases the sense of ownership.
- **Document the fun:** Take photos and videos! These become precious keepsakes.
- **Don't sweat perfection:** Things will go wrong, especially with little ones. The laughter when the cake falls apart becomes part of the tradition!
- **Let it evolve:** As kids get older, some traditions might lose their appeal. It's okay to phase things out or add new ones that better suit their interests.

Final Dad Thoughts

The traditions you start during those early years will shape your child's memories long after they're grown. It's kind of a big deal, but in the best possible way! Don't overthink it - just focus on creating moments of genuine connection, laughter, and love. Traditions are about presence, not presents. And that, dads, is something we're already experts at.

31. THE ROAD AHEAD: ONGOING JOYS AND CHALLENGES OF BEING A DAD

Alright, Dad. You've made it through the whirlwind of the first year. You've changed more diapers than you ever thought possible, survived some epic sleep deprivation, celebrated those incredible milestones, and maybe even shed a few happy tears along the way.

But guess what? The adventure has only just begun.

Being a dad isn't about crossing a finish line; it's about embracing a long and winding road. There will be joyous stretches, unexpected detours, maybe a few potholes along the way, but if you approach it with an open heart and a sense of humor, the journey is one of the most rewarding you'll ever take.

The Ever-Changing Landscape

Just when you think you've got a handle on things...BOOM! Your little guy undergoes yet another transformation. He's not just a squishy baby anymore. He's a toddler on the move, an inquisitive preschooler, a full-fledged kid ready for school. Each new phase brings its own set of incredible joys and, let's be honest, new challenges too.

Let's take a quick tour of what lies ahead:

- **The Toddler Years (Age 1-3):** Exploration mode is activated! They're walking, running, and discovering the world with a mix of excitement and the occasional tantrum. It's a time of big emotions, testing boundaries, and helping them navigate their ever-expanding world.

- **Preschool (Age 3-5):** This is where friendships blossom, imagination takes flight, and their personalities really shine. Get ready for endless questions, lots of playtime, and navigating social dynamics – theirs and yours at those playdates!

- **The Early School Years (Age 5-8):** Reading, writing, and (gulp) homework enter the picture. Suddenly, those baby snuggles are replaced with drop-off lines and helping them figure out how to be a good friend. And yes, you can still read them bedtime stories, even if the books get a lot longer.

Embrace the Shift

Your role as a dad continues to evolve as well. You're not just the diaper-changing, bottle-feeding superhero anymore. Now, you're a teacher, a guide, a confidante, and a role model. It's an awesome responsibility, but remember, you don't have to shoulder it alone. Lean on your partner, your own parents, friends and family, and all those resources you gathered in that first year.

Ongoing Joys You Can Count On

While every stage has its ups and downs, there's a certain magic that keeps drawing you deeper into your role as a dad. Here are just a few of those evergreen joys:

- **The Awe-Inspiring Moments:** It might be the first "I love you," their big grin after scoring a goal, or the way they beam with pride when you watch their school performance. Witnessing their growth is a constant source of amazement.

- **The Everyday Adventures:** The simple things become meaningful—trips to the park, bedtime stories, even building a pillow fort in the living room.

- **Your Bond:** The relationship you have with your child is unlike any other. Your hugs mean the world to them, even when they get big and act all preteen and cool.

The Inevitable Challenges (It's Okay, We're All in This Together)

Of course, there will also be bumps along the road. It's part of the deal. Here's a taste of what you might encounter:

- **Balancing Work and Dad-Life:** Finding that sweet spot and not feeling constantly pulled in different directions is an ongoing challenge.
- **Handling the Big Emotions:** Tantrums in toddlers, mood swings as they get older – sometimes it's as hard on us as it is on them. It's okay to take a parent time-out when you need one!
- **The Comparison Trap:** Don't fall for the Instagram-perfect parenting illusion. Every family has their messes, and we each find our own way to navigate those waters.

Advice from a Dad Who's Been There (Sort of)

Here are some things I wish I'd known earlier. I hope these bits of dad-wisdom help you on your journey:

- **Be present:** Put down the phone, get down on their level, and really connect. Those moments are precious and they pass faster than we realize.
- **It's okay to not be perfect:** No parent is. We all make mistakes, learn from them, and do better next time.

- **Find your tribe:** Having fellow dads you can lean on, laugh with, and share the real struggles with is priceless.
- **Don't forget about YOU:** Self-care isn't selfish. Whether it's squeezing in a workout, taking a hot shower, or having a laugh with friends, it makes you a better dad at the end of the day.

32. YOU'VE GOT THIS, DAD: REFLECTIONS ON YEAR ONE AND CELEBRATING YOUR JOURNEY

Okay, take a deep breath and grab some tissues because we're about to get a little sentimental here. You've made it! You've navigated spit-up, sleepless nights, first smiles, first steps, and all the incredible ups and downs in between.

Think back to the day your son was born. Remember those feelings – the excitement, the overwhelming love, and let's be honest, maybe just a hint of "Oh crap, what do I do now?"

That new dad holding his tiny baby might feel like a lifetime ago, but in another way, it was just yesterday. Look how far you've come!

Take a Victory Lap

Before we look to the future (and all the amazing adventures it holds), let's pause to celebrate all you've accomplished this year. Grab a notebook and a pen – it's time to reflect:

- **List those big milestones:** The first time your baby rolled over, crawled, said a word, walked...remember the pride that swelled up in your chest?
- **Recall the funny, everyday moments:** His goofy expressions, his obsession with a random toy, the way his eyes light up when you walk through the door.
- **Acknowledge your growth:** Think about all the diaper changes you've mastered, the bottles you've conquered, the sleep schedules you (somehow) survived. You're a baby-wrangling pro!
- **Give yourself some serious credit:** You've been there for the giggles and the cries. You've learned, you've adapted, and most importantly, you've loved this kid fiercely every step of the way. High five, Dad!

The Superhero You've Become

When you started this journey, you didn't have a cape or superpowers. What you did have was love for your son, and that, it turns out, is the greatest power of all. This past year has shaped you into a dad who is:

- **Stronger than you thought:** Not just physically (though hauling a car seat builds muscle!), but emotionally resilient. You've handled challenges with grace and determination.

- **More patient than you imagined:** Sure, there's still that moment when a diaper disaster strikes that tests your limits, but overall, you've gained a whole new level of patience.
- **Filled with joy in unexpected ways:** It's impossible to describe the feeling of pure love that fatherhood unlocks. Those little moments add up to a life overflowing with joy.

You may not feel like a superhero every day, especially when you're covered in food or running on fumes. But trust me, your son sees you as his hero.

The Journey Continues (But You're More Prepared!)

I'm not going to lie – there are more challenges ahead! Toddlerhood brings new adventures (and a whole new definition of "mess!)." But guess what? You're ready. Those basics you learned this past year? They're your foundation. You've got the confidence and the grit to handle whatever comes next.

Remember these truths as you go forth:

- **You're not alone:** Your partner, family, friends, and community – they're still your support squad. Lean on them when you need to.

- **Celebrate the good days:** Parenting will always have its tough moments, so make sure to relish those amazing days when things just click.
- **It's okay to make mistakes:** No dad is perfect, and that's okay! Learn from the missteps and keep showing up with love.
- **Have fun!:** Being a dad is the hardest job you'll ever love. Don't forget to find the pure joy in it – the goofy games, the bedtime stories, and the building of an unbreakable bond with your son.

A Message to My Son (For When You're Older)

Maybe someday, your son will read these words. If so, this part is for him.

[Son's name], watching you grow has been the greatest privilege of my life. You make me a better man each day. I hope you know that even when I messed up, I was always trying my best. I hope you feel fiercely loved, always supported, and ready to conquer the world with both strength and kindness.

You've Got This, Dad

Congratulations, Dad! You survived the wild and wonderful first year. Take a moment to breathe, to give yourself a big hug, and to bask in the incredible reality that you did it.

And now? Get ready for the next adventure! It's

going to be a blast.